KEYS TO UNDER- STANDING ALZHEIMER'S DISEASE

Dr. Gisèle P. Wolf-Klein
and Dr. Arnold P. Levy

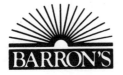

To our children, Liliane, Sophie, Lauren, and Brandon:
May they know a world where Alzheimer's disease is curable

Copyright © 1992 by Barron's Educational Series, Inc.

All inquiries should be addressed to:
Barron's Educational Series, Inc.
250 Wireless Boulevard
Hauppauge, New York 11788

Library of Congress Catalog Card No. 91-45174

International Standard Book No. 0-8120-4758-3

Library of Congress Cataloging-in-Publication Data

Wolf-Klein, Gisele P.
   Keys to understanding Alzheimer's disease / Gisele P. Wolf-Klein,
Arnold P. Levy.
      p. cm.—(Barron's retirement keys)
   Includes index.
   ISBN 0-8120-4758-3
   1. Alzheimer's disease—Popular works.   I. Levy, Arnold P.   II. Title.
III. Series.
RC523.2.W65   1991
616.8'31—dc20
                                   91-45174
                                      CIP

PRINTED IN THE UNITED STATES OF AMERICA
234   5500   987654321

CONTENTS

1

WHAT IS ALZHEIMER'S DISEASE?

Alzheimer's disease is characterized by "a progressive, global, cognitive loss." * In other words, when someone is afflicted with Alzheimer's disease, the mind is impaired and all intellectual functions worsen over time. The disease begins with a slow, barely perceptible loss of memory and evolves over many years into total mental incapacity. A *sudden change* in mental performance in an otherwise healthy adult is not Alzheimer's disease; such an obvious and abrupt change should prompt immediate medical attention. Similarly, an isolated episode of confusion that completely clears up is not Alzheimer's disease, but this too warrants further medical study to ascertain its cause and to apply appropriate treatment.

Memory loss is the hallmark of Alzheimer's disease, but our minds do much more than merely remember things. We think, assess, calculate, plan, judge, and decide. When a person develops Alzheimer's disease, he or she loses not only memory but also other areas of cognition, such as judgment and the ability to perform abstract reasoning. An example is the ability to balance a checkbook, which involves mathematical interpretation.

In a social setting, it is a common experience for all of us that a person approaches and, several times over the course of the conversation, repeats the same question. This individual has clearly forgotten not only that he or she asked the question in the first place but also your answer. There is obvious memory loss.

---

*American Psychiatric Association. *Diagnostic and Statistical Manual of Mental Disorders*. Third Edition. Washington, DC: American Psychiatric Press, 1987.

As we become involved in the conversation, we realize that there is more than loss of memory. The judgment is affected, too. The individual may make inappropriate comments. He or she may interrupt in the middle of the conversation, anxiously asking when will it be time to go home.

Consider, for instance, the successful Wall Street broker who is developing Alzheimer's disease. His family may have noticed memory lapses, but they assume he is distracted because he is such a busy man. He continues to go to work on a daily basis, but his job performance is now hindered by poor judgment. He may buy and sell stocks that are clearly inappropriate because he has lost the critical faculty to discern the value of the market. He might be unaware of his mistakes. It will take a series of mishaps and perhaps several complaints from trusted clients for company executives to realize he has a problem.

Disorders of speech and visual problems (reading a map and finding a location) may follow. The stockbroker can no longer find his way to an old college friend's home. He gets lost at an intersection and cannot remember whether to make a left or a right turn. When he checks the road map, he is no longer sure how to orient the map or how the map relates to his situation.

He may have difficulty finding words and may show frustration in the conversation. Little by little, he speaks less and isolates himself to avoid social contact. Usually the victim's physical condition, including the ability to walk, remains normal until late in the course of Alzheimer's disease. Eventually, however, the victim becomes bedridden, loses all brain function, and is unable to walk, to go to the toilet, or to eat unassisted.

When Alois Alzheimer originally described the disease in Germany in 1907, he reported the case of a 51-year-old woman. This individual was initially seen by the psychiatrist because of her strange behavior: she was agitated and jealous of her concerned and devoted husband. Shortly thereafter, her memory loss became apparent and her speech became impaired. She died five years later, bedridden and contracted in a fetal position.

Even though this was the first reported case of the disease, it is not a typical case of what we now recognize as Alzheimer's disease. Most Alzheimer's victims are 65 years of age and older, and the prevalence increases with age to one person in two over the age of 85. Women and men of all ethnic groups are affected. Individuals can live with this disease for over 10 years because they often remain physically healthy. At present, at least two and a half million people in the United States are afflicted with Alzheimer's disease.

The United States, like most of the Western world, is an aging society. Better technology and medical care keep elderly people alive longer. By the year 2030, 20 percent of the U.S. population will be over 65, compared to 12 percent today.

Khachaturian, a scientist at the U.S. National Institutes of Health, predicts that there might be over 14 million U.S. citizens with Alzheimer's disease by the year 2050. Because the illness is so common in later years, it is important for all of us to recognize possible early signs and to become familiar with the appropriate course of action, including current trends in research and community resources, such as support groups.

2

WHAT TO DO IF YOU SUSPECT YOU HAVE ALZHEIMER'S DISEASE

Don't panic!

One of our patients was convinced she suffered from Alzheimer's disease. As proof of her condition, she brought along several recent newspaper clippings on Alzheimer's disease, which she began to quote verbatim—from memory! Obviously, this person did not have the disease: she would have been unable to memorize complex and lengthy information. However, she expressed a natural and overwhelming concern for her decreased memory performance.

Many of us forget where we place our keys, what we were about to do, or the time of a dental appointment. In this frenetic world, it is easy to forget, but forgetting does not mean we have Alzheimer's disease.

First, it is perfectly normal to experience changes in memory with aging. The specific memory changes in normal aging are reviewed in Key 5. These changes do not reflect overall physical or intellectual performance: an 80-year-old orchestra conductor can remember a two hour musical score as well as and probably better than a 20-year-old student.

Second, there are many reasons that memory problems develop other than Alzheimer's disease. The most common cause is depression. With depression, one becomes unable to focus on matters to be remembered and is therefore unable to memorize them. For instance, we all experience memory problems when we are preoccupied with illness or money problems. Anxiety and nervousness can impair the memory process. This is not Alzheimer's disease.

The current opinion is that onset of depression late in life with no obvious precipitating cause should be investigated for underlying medical problems. In other words, people over the age of 65 who have been generally healthy, happy, and active and who lately find themselves more tearful and sad should consult a physician to see if there is a physical problem responsible for the feelings of depression.

Medical illnesses, such as thyroid imbalance, vitamin deficiencies, and small strokes, can cause memory problems. When multiple small strokes have occurred, the patient can have a pattern of memory loss very similar to the clinical picture of Alzheimer's disease. This is *multiinfarct dementia* (MID). The stroke may have been so small that the individual never noticed a physical problem, such as weakness of an arm or leg.

In fact, small strokes can sometimes complicate the picture of memory loss by combining their effects with the effect of coexisting Alzheimer's disease. The combined process can hasten the deterioration. When recognized and treated appropriately, these types of memory dysfunctions can improve.

Finally, many medications can cause impairment of memory. Good examples are cold medications, sleeping pills, or allergy remedies, which are all known to affect memory. Check all the medications you take, even those you "borrow" from your spouse or purchase over the counter. If you decide to consult a physician for memory loss, make sure that you bring along all these medications at the time of the office visit.

Third, even if you are in the very early stages of Alzheimer's disease, this is an illness that progresses slowly. Ahead are years of active and enjoyable life. In addition, a growing interest in research is now mounting and will, we hope, result in new therapies in the near future.

If you have been concerned about your memory performance or that of a loved one, seek medical advice *now* from an experienced physician (see Key 9). Do not sit home alone in a dark corner and brood over your unexpressed fears. Also, do not rely on the suggestions and opinions of your family or friends. They are not necessarily world experts on Alzheimer's disease. In addition, you will not be free to express all your concerns to loved ones because you may be embarrassed or afraid of burdening them with your problems. They in turn will not be unbiased in their evaluation because they may want to avoid hurting your feelings or frightening you by showing you the reality of what is happening. It is time for professional help.

3

STAGES OF ALZHEIMER'S DISEASE

The disease progresses over the course of years from an insidious start with occasional forgetfulness to an advanced bedridden state with total inability to speak (*aphasia*) in which the individual requires help with feeding, washing, and going to the toilet. The average survival period from the time of diagnosis to death is approximately 10 years. The speed of the deterioration process varies according to the individual. In some people, the process may take only a few years to reach the terminal stage. In others, it may last for 15 to 20 years.

There are basically three major phases of the disease. In the first stage, there is forgetfulness. This forgetfulness is usually obvious to close family members, but the individual continues to function in society and at work. In the second phase, the individual is more confused and anyone can notice that there is something wrong with his or her performance. Finally, in the advanced stage, the victim becomes totally incapacitated and cannot function without constant help. This is a very general description of the course of the disease; however, there are many individual variations as the victim progresses through these phases.

To facilitate the understanding of this process, several scientists have attempted to organize the clinical course into stages. The most commonly used systemization is the seven-stage description by Reisberg and his colleagues. This is the global deterioration scale of primary degenerative dementia (GDS). It is often used in medical publications to describe the state of the patients studied.

In the initial stage, there is no clear evidence of memory trouble and no cognitive decline. The individual performs well on psychometric tests, which are tests of mental function similar to those given to measure IQ. At this point, the individual is essentially normal.

The second stage shows only very mild memory problems, with difficulty in remembering names of friends. The changes at this point are still very subtle. The individual may continue to work, drive, and function in the community. Occasionally, a surprising statement might occur in the course of a conversation. For instance, the individual may inquire about the health of a friend who, everyone knows, died four years before. Only extensive psychometric testing would show a measurable change. In the second stage, except perhaps for a concerned spouse who may be wondering if there is something wrong, no one else is usually aware of the problem.

By the third stage, there is objective evidence of memory loss, which interferes with job performance. Some colleagues at work are becoming aware of the difficulties the person has in completing a task that used to be routine. The individual may be anxious and avoids social situations because he or she realizes that there is a problem.

In stage four, there is clinical evidence of memory impairment when objective mental status is tested by doctors. The disease is now becoming obvious to acquaintances as well as relatives and colleagues. Repetition is the hallmark of this stage, rendering daily companionship more difficult. The spouse and children are becoming increasingly frustrated and upset as the afflicted individual cannot remember information. A common pattern of conversation—What are we going to eat tonight? Chicken and string beans—is repeated several times at 10 minute intervals until the exasperated spouse explodes, "I told you twenty times already!"

Although in stage four the family is becoming more burdened, the victim often becomes less anxious and depressed as his or her feelings are dulled and judgment decreases.

Stage five shows problems with both recent and past memories and with recalling events pertinent to close family members, such as birthdays, friendships, and interests. Judgment is failing; the individual is no longer able to select appropriate clothes for the season or to match items by colors. The caring grandmother brings her young grandchildren presents that are not safe for their age.

Eventually, the victim of Alzheimer's disease may leave the water running, the stove on, or the front door open. At this point wandering becomes a major problem. The individual is not sure that he or she belongs in the once familiar surroundings of the home and attempts to leave. The victim is disoriented in time and place and cannot answer the question, "What year is it?"

In stage six, comprehension of language diminishes and simple commands are not understood. Victims may revert to the language of childhood, if English is a second language. Eventually, language disappears altogether, other intellectual abilities deteriorate, and the victim becomes incoherent. Assistance in the care of the individual becomes mandatory because the spouse must get some respite to avoid burnout.

In the terminal stage, or stage seven, the victim becomes bedridden and totally dependent for all functions. He or she is incontinent of urine and feces, can no longer speak intelligibly, and cannot eat unassisted. Death usually results from *aspiration pneumonia*, pneumonia caused by breathing in food or other objects because the victim does not remember how to swallow food safely, or from overwhelming urinary infections.

The speed at which sufferers from Alzheimer's disease move from one stage to the next varies greatly from one individual to another. Also, the individual's personality affects general behavior throughout the illness. A gentle, soft-spoken person may continue to behave very pleasantly despite advanced dementia. Sometimes individuals may also go through periods of agitation, requiring medications, and then reverse through stages of peacefulness, when they need only supervision and quiet guidance.

As a family member, you are a key person. Often, you are the one who first notices subtle changes in memory and in behavior. You are the one who can decide to seek medical advice. You are the one who can present your observations to the doctor and describe examples of memory loss, length of symptoms, and existence of potentially important life events that may lately have disrupted your loved one's existence and contributed to depression. It is with your help that the physician will come up with the correct diagnosis and the appropriate management of behavioral symptoms.

4

WHAT CAUSES ALZHEIMER'S DISEASE?

When Alzheimer first described the disease in 1907, he included in his presentation a report of the brain autopsy. He was struck by the marked changes in the structure of the brain nerve cells. These cells had disappeared in many places, leaving tangles of fibrous tissue. He also noted the deposition of a "peculiar substance in the cerebral cortex."

Today, microscopic examination of the brain of Alzheimer's patients has not revealed much more than Alzheimer himself saw. Brain cells die. In their place, two abnormal findings are typical: the plaques and the tangles. These include remnants of the original healthy nerve cells; they are still made of protein but are very altered. The agent responsible for the alteration in the protein, leading to the loss of the complex architecture of nerve cells, is unknown at this point.

However, some progress has been made in understanding the nature of the altered protein. The plaques appear to be made of a component called beta-amyloid, which seems to proliferate in Alzheimer's disease and destroys the normal structure of the brain cell. The beta-amyloid protein kills the normal nerve cell, but its toxicity can be stopped by a chemical called substance P, which was described by Yankner in 1990. In an exciting study, he found that rats injected with the beta-amyloid substance forgot what they had recently learned. Rats injected with substance P were protected; they did not develop memory problems. It seems that the amyloid protein itself causes memory troubles. Amyloid can also be seen in the brain of elderly people who do not have Alzheimer's disease and is not necessarily the exclusive source of the disease.

11

Another key protein found in normal brains is the tau protein, which physically links brain cells through microtubules, allowing communication and transport of biological molecules. The tau protein is damaged by the Alzheimer's process and communication is lost. Large agglomerates of the damaged tau protein become part of the tangles, the evidence of dying brain cells. The factors responsible for this damage remain unknown.

In trying to understand why brain cells die in Alzheimer's disease, research efforts have focused on discovering factors that interfere with normal protein function in the brain.

Besides the alteration in the protein components, there seems to be a lack of balance of *excitatory function* (stimulation) and *inhibitory function* (restraining) of the brain cells. Cells in general achieve a delicate electrical balance by maintaining the amount of chemical compounds such as sodium and potassium inside their membranes. When cells are stimulated or excited, electrical activity occurs that can be measured. This is how electrocardiograms are recorded. The same electrical activity occurs in brain cells, where electroencephalograms can show the activity of various parts of the brain. At the level of the brain cell, too much stimulation could result in brain cell death. These findings have led to new theories that concern the role of glutamic and aspartic acids. These are amino acids that may overstimulate the nerve cell under abnormal or disease conditions.

A very recent discovery pertains to the role of nitric oxide, which may moderate cell function by playing the role of a messenger. Nitric oxide is a simple and common gas produced constantly during the natural process of the body's metabolism. It may be used by cells to kill bacteria that have invaded the system. Nitric oxide is implicated in the degenerative process of many neurological maladies, from Huntington's disease to Alzheimer's disease. Other theories pertaining to Alzheimer's disease are based on the potential role of aluminum and other so-called toxins (see Key 13).

Some dementing illnesses have been attributed to the existence of a "slow virus," which may take years to produce disease. For instance, epidemics of unexplained behavior in cattle in the United Kingdom have been linked to the consumption of infected feed made from virus-contaminated bone meal. In humans, Creutzfeldt and Jakob described a progressive deterioration of mental and physical functioning caused by a slowly acting virus. A similar illness, *kuru* (trembling with fear), was found in New Guinea, where natives consumed human organs contaminated by viruses, such as the brain, bone marrow, and viscera. There is no evidence at this point that Alzheimer's disease is of infectious origin.

The role of genetic transmission is not completely understood at this time (see Key 7). Here again, however, there is little evidence to support heredity as a major factor in most forms of Alzheimer's disease.

The causes of Alzheimer's disease are probably multiple. Clearly, some physical and chemical alterations in the brain cells have been recognized and identified. Beta-amyloid protein destroys the normal structure of the brain and is certainly responsible for some of the changes seen in Alzheimer's disease. Future research in various medical fields should explain these causes and point the way to corrective and, we hope, curative and preventive treatment.

5

MEMORY CHANGES IN NORMAL AGING

As mentioned in Key 1, memory loss is the hallmark of Alzheimer's disease. Memory changes can also be seen in normal nondemented elderly people, however. Therefore, not all memory lapses should be attributed to a pathological process. In this key, we review those memory changes seen in normal aging.

Memory is a complex function that can be simplified into four separate and sequential steps:

Sensory memory   primary memory (short-term)
secondary memory (long-term)   tertiary memory (permanent)

Let us observe the tourist who goes to a museum to view a special collection of famous impressionist paintings. He ambles into the first gallery, glances around, and sees some old Italian masterworks from the fifteenth century.

Not finding these to be of particular interest, he moves to the next gallery, where he happens upon the modern style he has come to see. He looks at the paintings: his sensory memory is visually activated and awakens a desire to learn more.

The tourist now selects a specific painting he really likes. He studies the composition, observes the contours, and marvels at the contrast of colors: he is transferring the information from sensory memory to primary short-term memory.

At this point, he is at great risk of forgetting this wonderful painting, unless he processes the freshly acquired information into the secondary, long-term memory by thoroughly studying all the details he has recently noted. This can be achieved by sketching the painting on a pad, by writing down the name of the artist and perhaps the date of the painting, by discussing with a companion the selection of colors, and by purchasing a postcard or a good reproduction that can be looked at later.

Finally, after many practice sessions, such as showing slides of the painting to friends and family members, the information is stored into tertiary memory and becomes part of his permanent knowledge.

With normal aging, only sensory information and secondary memory are affected. *Primary* and *tertiary* memory remain normal even with advancing years, so that most elderly people enjoy sharing information stored long ago, to the delight of their grandchildren!

- Sensory information, the first step in the memory process, can be impaired because of visual or hearing loss. After all, one cannot be expected to remember something that was not seen or heard! These losses should be recognized and corrected with proper eyeglasses or hearing aid devices.

- Research has shown that aging in itself causes problems with the secondary memory. Organizing the material to be remembered and retrieving the information speedily becomes impaired in normal aging: it's difficult to remember on the spur of the moment the name of someone or someplace, but the information is not forgotten, and it will probably come back—at 2 in the morning! Fortunately, this normal aging impairment can be reversed by using memory tricks, called *mnemonics*. These tricks have been known for many, many years and are used every day by professional "memory" people, such as actors and politicians. The great Roman orator Cicero used to remember his speeches by picturing himself in his own house, moving from one room to the other in a logical sequence as he would move from one paragraph to the next, linking his train of thought. In a similar fashion, one can better remember items on a shopping list if these items are organized into a logical sequence, associated with mental pictures, or arranged into a funny sentence. Advertising agencies use rhyming jingles to impress on our sensory memory the message they wish to sell.

As a rule, elderly people can function very well in life and can remember most important facts. In fact, they often learn to organize their life to compensate for occasional memory lapses by using shopping lists or diaries. Many children or young adults who have not yet learned to use these coping skills are much more "forgetful" than their elders!

6

MEMORY LOSS IN ALZHEIMER'S DISEASE

There is now strong evidence that all four steps of the normal memory process (see Key 5) are affected in Alzheimer's disease.

Sensory memory cannot process information because of a lack of attention span or general interest in trying to remember, and perhaps also a lack of understanding of the need to comply with the task required. For instance, suppose that our museum tourist in Key 5 is now affected with Alzheimer's disease. He does not remember the famous impressionist painting because by the time he reaches the second gallery he has actually lost interest in looking at the painting he came to see in the first place.

Researchers have tested **primary memory** (which is preserved in normal aging) in Alzheimer's disease. Subjects are given a list of names or numbers to repeat immediately. They cannot comply with this task well. They forget several items on the list, and they show a progressive decrease in the number of words or numbers they can remember as the disease evolves.

Secondary memory, which can be impaired in normal aging, also shows in Alzheimer's disease a deterioration in the recall as well as recognition of words or objects.

Finally, **tertiary memory** may appear to be preserved: these individuals talk about events from childhood. When nondemented siblings or friends of the same generation participate in the conversation, however, it becomes clear that these events are not accurately remembered. The description of the childhood home is incorrect. Names of teachers or college friends are mixed up.

How can we recognize these four complex and now impaired steps of memory in the Alzheimer's victim? At first, the memory loss is subtle and slight, progressing slowly. Mrs. L.C., a 72-year-old woman, is going to lunch with a good friend of hers. En route to the restaurant, they pass in front of a bakery, which reminds Mrs. L.C. of a funny story. As she recounts the story to her friend, they have a good laugh about it and proceed on with their walk. After lunch, on the way home, passing in front of the same bakery, Mrs. L.C. repeats the identical story to her friend, not remembering that she did so only a short time before on the way to the restaurant. This incident suggests memory trouble in the otherwise healthy Mrs. L.C.

Sometimes these memory changes are so subtle that family and friends do not notice them. For example, a nondemented spouse might spontaneously take over the tasks that are no longer properly being done by the affected spouse without being aware of it. The dishes are washed, the beds are made, and the house seems to be in order when friends come to visit. Only a disruptive event, such as the illness, hospitalization, or travel of the nondemented spouse, reveals the problem: the afflicted individual cannot prepare a meal or find the right clothes without someone's help.

The memory loss that is evident when people repeat the same story or ask the same questions at short intervals extends itself eventually to failure of judgment. These individuals can no longer balance checkbooks or deal with other financial matters. They cannot continue to perform at work or in social gatherings. As the present becomes more difficult to remember, they seek refuge in the past. Eventually, even the past disappears, as Alzheimer's victims forget where they are and who they are.

7

ROLE OF HEREDITY

When someone in your family develops Alzheimer's disease, a natural concern is raised: Is it hereditary? What are my chances of developing the same illness Dad seems to have? The thought that Alzheimer's disease might have a genetic component is not new.

In 1926, Meggendorfer referred to the concept of "familial Alzheimer's disease." Since then, several other scientists have sought families with a high occurrence of memory troubles. Unfortunately, it is extremely difficult to establish with certainty a genetic tree of Alzheimer's disease because ancestors with "senility" may not have been diagnosed accurately; they may have actually suffered from other psychiatric illnesses or vascular disease (such as hardening of the arteries). In addition, many ancestors may have died at an early age, without having lived long enough to develop the disease. Another problem for researchers is to find reliable sources of information over 100 years old. Before the nineteenth century, the only relatively common information on families were parish books, which are very difficult to read and interpret.

Now, however, for a few well-established families in England, Holland, and Italy, the documented prevalence of Alzheimer's disease is very high, affecting members of each generation. Several centers in the United States have identified a handful of families with a high incidence of Alzheimer's disease. Obviously, these families are closely scrutinized and monitored by scientists. It appears that Alzheimer's disease in these families occurs at an earlier age. For instance, a family going back to the middle of the eighteenth century has been identified and studied in Calabria, Italy. Of 6000 people, 61 are known to have had signs of early Alzheimer's disease (average age of onset was 42). These 61 people are thought to have a common ancestor, a woman born in 1715 who lived until the age of 45.

These families probably suffer from a type of Alzheimer's disease that is a distinct genetic form. In these large families, the disorder affects every generation, males and females, and the children have a 50 percent chance of developing the disease. This is *autosomal dominant inheritance*, which means that the transmission occurs directly from parent to child.

A British researcher, St. George Hyslop, identified in 1987 a familial Alzheimer's disease (FAD) gene located on chromosome 21. Abnormalities in this chromosome were already recognized as responsible for Down's syndrome. Indeed, it appears that patients with Down's syndrome frequently develop Alzheimer's disease toward the end of their short lives, around the age of 35. The relationship between Alzheimer's disease and Down's syndrome supports the hypothesis that in some cases Alzheimer's disease is linked to a genetic cause. How often and to what degree remain unclear. Not all patients with Down's syndrome develop Alzheimer's disease at the end of their lives, and the large majority of patients with Alzheimer's disease do not have Down's syndrome. In fact, it is quite possible that more than one gene is involved in Alzheimer's disease.

Another way to explore the role of genetics in the transmission of diseases is to study *identical twins*, who are born with exactly the same genes, and to find out how often one twin develops the same illness as the other. If the illness is transmitted through the genes, then both twins should eventually have the same malady. Nee and Polinsky studied 22 twin pairs referred to the National Institutes of Health. Only 40 percent of these twin siblings of Alzheimer's victims ultimately developed the disease.

These statistics are inconclusive in supporting the genetic transmission of Alzheimer's disease. Alzheimer's disease may be a *heterogeneous* disease: some forms are more readily transmitted genetically than others. By establishing closely monitored *pedigrees* of families (family trees); we will learn more about familial Alzheimer's disease. There is no compelling evidence at present to support the idea that most forms of Alzheimer's disease are hereditary and will be transmitted from parents to children.

8

SO YOU HAVE ALZHEIMER'S DISEASE—NOW WHAT?

If your doctor has recently diagnosed your memory loss as probably due to Alzheimer's disease, you are now distressed and worried. Many questions come to your mind.

How long do I have to live?

Be assured that Alzheimer's disease is usually a slowly progressive disease that will take 10 to 15 years to develop fully, although the disease can progress faster in some individuals. It is sometimes difficult to know exactly when the disease started. As a rule, however, this is an illness that is measured in years, not months.

Will I have any physical pain?

Chances are you have developed this disease in your 70s or 80s. No physical pain is associated with it. In fact, elderly people affected by this disease generally remain unusually physically healthy for their age. In our clinical experience, the common illnesses encountered with aging, such as heart disease, cancer, and arthritis, seem to spare the Alzheimer's patient. However, some mental distress and depression are usually associated with Alzheimer's disease, particularly in the early stage, when you may be more aware of memory loss. This is the time to see your physician and seek treatment for depression.

Will I know I am getting worse?

If you reach the very advanced stages of the illness, you will not be aware of it and you are not likely to suffer from it. Your family will be burdened and you can take measures now to help them later. Think about what will happen to your family if you become bedridden. Discuss with them what you would want done for you later, when you can no longer make decisions for yourself.

What should I do now?

Plan now for the future. Arrange your finances, and seek legal counseling. Remember, your memory may be failing but your judgment and decision-making processes are still good.

Check your personal records. You should have on file your name and social security number and the addresses of all immediate family and friends you would like to contact, the location of your will or trust, your religious affiliation with the name of a chaplain, rabbi, or priest if appropriate, the name of your doctors, lawyers, and other key professional people, and a request or your arrangements for burial. Your financial records should list banks, sources of income, and assets, such as retirement money, checking account, and insurance information. If you have a mortgage, debts, or credits, list them.

Be aware that most health insurance agencies do not cover chronic illnesses like Alzheimer's disease. Medicare does not pay for long-term care in a nursing home. Do you want to go to a nursing home, or would you rather have home health care? Will you want to proceed with a living will, health care proxy, and do not resuscitate guidelines (see Key 48)? Hospitals now require patient self-determination advance guidelines directives before you can be admitted. They want to know what *you* want them to do for you.

Will I transmit the illness to my children?

You might be concerned for your children. Is this illness hereditary? The answer is, probably not, at least not in a dominant pattern, that is, from parent to child. Also, research in this area is growing and chances are that there will be an effective treatment by the time your children reach a susceptible age.

What can I do for myself today?

Above all, focus on the *quality* of your life for the next few years, not the quantity. You will probably remain physically healthy and able to enjoy physical activity. Develop a program of gentle and regular exercise, eat good-tasting, nutritious meals, and have regular checkups to prevent or control other medical illnesses. Recent studies have shown that walking at least 20 minutes a day, preferably in the fresh air, is beneficial to Alzheimer's victims.

Rearrange your life to make it fit your current and future needs. Call friends and family members whom you haven't contacted in many years. Now is the time to get over old family quarrels. If you have put off a trip you wanted to take but never had time for, go ahead and do it. Celebrate life today, because you can enjoy the present.

You may want to consider short-term psychotherapy to discuss and ventilate your concerns and your anxieties and maybe deal with early depression. Don't expect your spouse or your children to listen to and accept all your feelings.

Plan your retirement now, and hire appropriate help. Look for good caretakers. Speak to your friends and relatives about people they might know who would be willing to work for you. Tell your relatives what to expect in clear, simple words: My doctor said I have Alzheimer's disease, so I might not remember things you tell me. Be aware that you may become unduly suspicious of family and friends. Share this with your loved one, who may otherwise become devastated by false accusations.

Consider enrolling yourself in a research study at the local university. Contact the medical department of the university, and ask if they are conducting research on Alzheimer's disease. You can also contact the Alzheimer's Disease Education and Referral Center (301-495-3311) for the name of the nearest Alzheimer's Disease Center and Satellite Diagnostic and Treatment Clinics.

9

HOW TO FIND A PHYSICIAN WITH EXPERTISE IN ALZHEIMER'S DISEASE

There are four groups of physicians who can help you in dealing with Alzheimer's disease: (1) psychiatrists, (2) neurologists, (3) internists and family practitioners, and (4) geriatricians.

The Psychiatrist

Traditionally, memory changes were attributed to aging and often referred to as "senility." When these changes were accompanied by other mental symptoms, such as agitation or hallucinations, patients were brought to psychiatrists. Indeed, for the 80 years since the initial description of Alzheimer's disease by the German psychiatrist Alois Alzheimer, the study and the research of "brain" illnesses has been the domain of psychiatry.

Today the psychiatrist often remains a key member of the medical team to help the victim and the family recognize and accept the disease, as well as to treat occasional behavioral manifestations. The psychiatrist is helpful not only in diagnosing the Alzheimer's disease but also in dealing with the array of feelings from both the victim and the family: fear, denial, anger, guilt, depression, and hope. Often, the earliest presentation of Alzheimer's disease is a subtle change in the individual's attitude and mood. Even before family members realize that there is memory loss, the individual is aware that he or she is not functioning as well as before.

Mood alterations are very common and disquieting to the victim and family. The psychiatrist can explain and treat the symptoms observed. As new behavioral symptoms appear, the psychiatrist becomes a critical and essential support to the family in explaining the expected mood changes and reassuring families as well as helping families to avoid overreacting.

The Neurologist

Neurologists, physicians who specialize in the function of the nervous system, including the brain, have also studied Alzheimer's disease and its impact on cognitive function. They are able to accurately diagnose the illness and to provide insight into the expected course and prognosis. Neurologists may be particularly helpful if you or your physician suspects that the individual may have multiinfarct dementia as a result of a series of strokes (see Key 2).

Internists and Family Practitioners

With growing public awareness of Alzheimer's disease as a major health issue, an extraordinary effort has been undertaken to educate and interest medical practitioners other than specialists in the brain and nervous system. Internists and family practitioners have learned to score *baseline* (before disease) memory performance in routine testing using simple *cognitive* (related to knowledge, both awareness and judgment) scales. They have also learned to search for reversible medical causes of memory problems, to rule out these causes before Alzheimer's is considered.

If you do not know of a good internist, family practitioner, neurologist, or psychiatrist, you can call a nearby referral hospital and ask for the name and telephone number of a consultant who is knowledgeable about Alzheimer's disease. Ask the operator or receptionist to be connected to the medical department. Medical secretaries usually have lists of consultants they are glad to share with you.

When you telephone the doctor's office, ask whether he or she is familiar with and interested in Alzheimer's disease before you make an appointment. This saves you time and money.

The Geriatrician

Recently, a new breed of physicians concerned specifically with the needs of elderly people has emerged. They are called geriatricians. Because Alzheimer's disease is a major issue in geriatric medicine, all trained geriatricians can test for memory changes, outline the most likely causes, treat symptoms, and provide support to the victim and family. A new subspecialty medical board in geriatrics was created in 1988. An updated list of certified geriatricians in your area can be obtained by calling the American Geriatrics Society (212-308-1414).

10

OFFICE EVALUATION OF THE ALZHEIMER'S VICTIM

Time of the Appointment

When you call the doctor's office to make the appointment for the initial visit, schedule it at a time when the Alzheimer's sufferer is less likely to be agitated and when you know that you will have enough time to get him or her ready without pressure. A late morning appointment, between 10 and 11 A.M., is usually best. In general, you are better off waiting a few days for a convenient appointment time rather than rushing in the next day unless the timing is good for both you and the sick person. Evening appointments are a particularly poor choice of timing because agitation is often worse in the Alzheimer's victim as night approaches. Also, ask the secretary when you are least likely to have to wait for a long period of time. Explain the situation. Neither the secretary nor you wants to keep an agitated individual waiting!

Ask whether you should feed the individual before the visit or whether the doctor expects him or her to be fasting for a blood test. If the individual should be fasting, be sure to pack a sandwich or cookies, which you can give your loved one as soon as the blood is drawn. While you have the secretary on the phone, find out what the doctor's fees are and whether Medicare assignment is accepted.

Getting to the Doctor's Office

There is no need to alert your loved one in advance of the doctor's appointment. The idea may be very frightening and disturbing, and it is likely that he or she will forget this information shortly thereafter. It is better to proceed with the normal daily routine of getting dressed and walking to the car. It is usually helpful to ask a family member or a friend to accompany you if parking the car is a problem. When you are ready to leave for the appointment, just tell the Alzheimer's victim that you are both going. Do not ask questions—Do you want to go? or Are you ready to go?—because you might meet with opposition, which leads to confrontation.

Many spouses find it helpful to explain the purpose of the medical visit by stating that they themselves need to see the doctor for their own health, which is actually true.

Whom to Take Along

When you arrive at the doctor's office for the first visit, make sure that the caregiver, that is, the person most closely associated with the Alzheimer's victim's daily activities, is present. This person may be yourself, the spouse, a child, a homemaker, or a friend.

The first essential part of the office evaluation is to obtain a comprehensive history from someone who knows the individual well, preferably someone who has observed the individual over a long period of time. The doctor is likely to ask for early signs of memory *dysfunction* (abnormality) in an attempt to accurately date the onset of the illness and to assess its progression. Think back: when was the first time you noticed something was wrong?

Also, bring along all medications, including over-the-counter drugs, used in the past year. Do not forget medical reports and x-rays.

How to Prepare the Individual Physically

During the physical examination, the physician will want to assess the individual's general presentation, including personal hygiene. It is quite commendable for the caregiver to attempt to thoroughly bathe and dress the individual before the visit, but this procedure may be distressing to the individual and misleading to the physician. To the extent possible, the individual should be allowed to wash, dress, groom, and apply makeup as he or she would do normally. Poor general hygiene is not a reflection of your care but rather a solid indicator of the individual's performance of the tasks of daily life.

Make sure that you choose comfortable clothes that are easy to put on and to remove. Avoid layers of underwear unless the weather is extraordinarily cold. The best choice is usually a jogging suit, which can be pulled up or down very quickly, making the examination easy to perform and non-threatening to the individual. Avoid high-heeled shoes for women, which are always hazardous but can be particularly dangerous if the individual is nervous and agitated.

Do not plan much on the day of the first visit. You should not be under pressure to leave the doctor's for another appointment, for example. The Alzheimer's victim may perceive your stress and become more agitated. Before you leave the office, find out how you can reach the doctor in an emergency and what other support services are suggested at this point.

11

TESTS FOR COGNITIVE FUNCTION AND ALZHEIMER'S DISEASE

Because the clinical picture of Alzheimer's disease is now well described, physicians can arrive at the correct diagnosis with accuracy in almost 90 percent of the cases. Only a brain biopsy during the victim's life or an autopsy after death can guarantee the correct diagnosis in every case. To help the physician make the diagnosis, several tests are performed. Unfortunately, there is not yet a characteristic marker for Alzheimer's disease that can be easily identified in the blood, although at this time several researchers appear to be on the verge of discovering one.

Standard Blood Work

The physician will order standard blood work to eliminate other possible causes for dementia, such as a problem of the thyroid gland or a vitamin deficiency. Two to three small tubes of blood are drawn for this purpose from the arm. Blood drawing is practically painless and has no serious risks. It is important to remember that one cannot develop AIDS from puncture with a clean sterilized needle and syringe.

Mental Function Testing in the Office

The doctor will want to obtain a baseline score of mental performance. Many tests have been described and are very helpful in "scoring" the degree of impairment, although none can make the definite diagnosis of Alzheimer's disease. One of the most commonly used tests is the mini-mental status examination (MMSE), described in 1976 by Folstein and his colleagues. This test asks a series of questions on the day's date, the location of the examination, the recall of objects, mathematical agility, such as subtraction, and simple commands. The maximum score is 30. A score below 20 supports the diagnosis of brain dysfunction. Another test that has recently received much attention is the clock drawing test. Patients who are unable to correctly place numbers in a circle representing a clock are likely to have some degree of dementia. Most of these mental tests meant to be given in the office are short, which makes them very useful in testing people with short attention spans.

Neuropsychological Testing

Some doctors may recommend comprehensive neuropsychological testing. This is a complex battery of tests administered by a neuropsychologist, usually over two sessions of one to two hours each. Individuals may be asked to repeat a succession of numbers or words, to recall a story, or to recognize faces. Each of these tasks requires that a specific part of the brain function properly. The neuropsychologist can then locate the site of the brain most affected by the disease. The cost of this testing is usually high, averaging $300. Your Medicare insurance will probably cover 80 percent of the expenses.

Brain Imaging

Most physicians suggest that the individual suspected of having Alzheimer's disease undergo brain imaging, that is, a radiological examination to look at the structure of the brain. The purpose is to rule out other possible causes for brain dysfunction, such as a brain tumor or *vascular lesions* (blood vessel injuries) as a result of strokes.

There are several ways of getting a good picture of the brain. Currently, we use the CAT scan (computerized axial tomography) or MRI (magnetic resonance imaging). Both are accurate and helpful. The CAT scan still uses radiation, whereas the MRI technology uses magnetic forces. For this reason, the MRI cannot be used in people with pacemakers. The CAT scan takes approximately 30 minutes; the MRI can take up to one hour. Also, the MRI is performed in a rather claustrophobic environment with a large machine surrounding the subject's head. The procedure, although not physically uncomfortable, may be anxiety provoking. Sedation is sometimes required. The cost of a CAT scan averages $400, whereas the cost of an MRI can be up to $900. Medicare currently reimburses 80 percent of these fees.

Newer approaches to brain imaging are the PET and SPECT scans: they provide an image of the function of the brain in addition to its structure (see also Key 12). They are used to study the metabolism of the brain, that is, the way the brain utilizes nutrients, such as glucose. It is known that in Alzheimer's disease there is decreased activity of the brain cells located in the *temporoparietal areas*, those areas of the brain located above the ears on the sides of the head. Decreased activity on a PET scan or SPECT scan in these areas supports the clinical diagnosis of Alzheimer's disease, as opposed to other dementing illnesses, which usually affect different parts of the brain.

PET studies are used strictly in research at this point. They are extremely expensive, over $2000 per study. The SPECT scan is cheaper and will probably become more widely available to medical doctors. Its use remains to be established.

12

ROLE OF NUTRITION

Good nutrition is a key to the proper management of Alzheimer's disease. Feeding the Alzheimer's victim is a real challenge, however. Many caregivers report that these individuals have voracious appetites and eat nonstop if offered food. An Alzheimer's victim returning from a restaurant might ask his companion, "When are we going to eat?" This behavior creates confusion in the mind of the caregiver and sometimes guilt and anger. Should I prepare and serve another full meal, after having just finished the last meal? Should I ignore him? Should I buy him a quick snack? There is also a feeling of unappreciation for the caregiver's work, which can be summarized by, Whatever I do, it's never enough.

Let us try to understand the process of nutrition for the Alzheimer's victim. Like anyone else, these individuals need protein, fat, and carbohydrates. By the age of 65, the average amount of calories needed decreases to anywhere between 1200 and 1600 calories per day depending on the individual level of activity. However, it is possible that Alzheimer's victims may require higher amounts of calories. Several studies have demonstrated increased food intake and yet reported weight loss. One of these studies, completed in Sweden in 1987, mentioned that patients were eating over 2000 calories per day! It is not clear today whether this increased caloric requirement is a result of increased activity, such as pacing, rocking, and abnormal motions, or whether there might be a true hyperactive metabolic state like that seen in patients with a very active thyroid gland.

For insight into brain metabolism, researchers are now using an advanced techology called positron emission tomography (PET) scan. This new technology allows us to visualize the function of the brain. The procedure studies the consumption of glucose, the essential fuel of brain cells, by the body. With this radiological technique, we know that glucose is not well utilized in certain areas of the brain affected by Alzheimer's disease. Is this because affected brain cells are dead and can no longer consume glucose, or is it that the glucose cannot get to the brain cells? The answer to this fundamental question may provide new leads in the therapy of the disease.

Some Alzheimer's sufferers also seem to have sweet cravings, choosing to consume large quantities of ice cream and cookies. They may need the glucose contained in these foods, or they may be reaching for the immediate and pleasant reward of a "treat." Psychiatrists are often confronted with hostile and aggressive patients in the emergency room. A quick approach consists of feeding them carbohydrates, such as cookies, which calms them.

In summary, our personal experience is that food restriction in the individual with Alzheimer's disease is not beneficial and may in fact be counterproductive. Those well-meaning spouses who attempt to impose their own diabetic diet, with artificial sweeteners and low-calorie foods, may actually deprive the individual of necessary nutrients. Three nutritious meals of at least 400 calories and preferably two additional snacks of high-energy nutrients should provide enough caloric intake to meet the needs of these active individuals. A judicious selection of proteins, cereals, fruits, and vegetables using fresh ingredients whenever possible is the best option. Remember that finger foods are often easier for both victim and caregiver to handle in the moderate to advanced stages of the disease. Chicken nuggets, meatballs, and fishcakes (without bones!) are ideal protein choices. Vegetables can be prepared in a puree to be eaten with a spoon. Be careful with grapes; it is easy to choke on them. Instead, provide peeled slices of grapefruit or orange.

If the individual forgets that she just ate and asks for more food, give her some! You may want to freeze and store meal portions that can be heated quickly, reducing your level of frustration when your loved one wants food *now*. Also, carry nutritious cookies that can be given to the Alzheimer's victim outdoors, in shopping malls, or at the doctor's office.

As the disease progresses, feeding the Alzheimer's victim becomes more difficult. They have forgotten how to ask for food, where to get it, and how to eat. Continue to prepare at least three meals a day, involving the individual as much as possible in the preparation of these meals. For instance, you may want to bake a batch of cookies or reheat rolls or bread in the oven to provide the lovely aroma of baked goods.

If food becomes stuck in a person's mouth because he forgot to swallow, give him some water to drink. Liquid may encourage the swallowing mechanism. Sometimes stroking the cheek or the throat very lightly may help.

Toward the end of the disease, the individual may no longer be able to eat. He or she may start choking on food. At this point, it is time to consider whether you want to supply nutrition by tube feeding. Food is given through a small plastic tube inserted either through the nose (nasogastric tube—NG tube) or directly into the stomach (PEG tube). An NG tube can be inserted at the bedside by any health professional with expertise. Often a visiting nurse can replace the tube at home. A PEG tube requires the skills of a gastroenterologist or a surgeon, who makes a small incision, under local anesthesia, in the skin covering the stomach. This is a benign procedure with very minimal risk, but it is a surgical intervention. The advantage is that PEG tubes are often less disruptive to the patient, who thus is less likely to pull them out. They are also esthetically more pleasing, which is important if you expect young visitors at the bedside. A regular intravenous tube can supply only fluid but not enough calories and nutrients to keep someone alive after a few weeks. Special feedings are sometimes given for short periods of time through the veins, but these feedings must be prepared very carefully to avoid the risk of infection. They require an expert team of medical professionals, which most nursing homes do not have. These feedings are not appropriate for the chronic nutritional requirements of the patient with Alzheimer's disease.

The decision to feed by tube is up to the victim and the caregiver (see Key 48). The decision is always difficult and sometimes traumatic. Discuss this process well in advance with the physician.

Key issues to keep in mind as you consider artificial feeding are as follows:

1. Would the patient have wanted it?
2. Will this treatment be successful, that is, prevent further weight loss and malnutrition?
3. Are the benefits of this treatment worth the possible problems, such as discomfort in inserting the tube, requirement for hand restraints to avoid having the patient pull out the tube, or local skin irritation at the site of the tube?

Nobody has the answers to all these questions, but you will feel more at peace if you have given at least some serious thought to these issues, before starting to feed by tube. Remember that many staff members and nursing home administrators become very uncomfortable with the decision to discontinue tube feeding once it has been started. Talk to health care professionals, get the physician's advice, and ask the nurse's opinion. Visit other patients who are fed by tube and ask their caregivers how they made their decision.

13

ROLE OF ALUMINUM AND OTHER TOXINS

Considerable excitement occurred when high levels of aluminum were found in the brains of individuals with Alzheimer's disease. However, no one knows whether this toxin is the cause, the consequence, or an additional factor in the development of Alzheimer's disease. For instance, aluminum is also found in patients with advanced renal failure who are undergoing dialysis.

The scientific world is still divided on the role of aluminum in the development of Alzheimer's. Until further proof of aluminum's dangers is found, it is wise to avoid excessive use of the product. For example, use non-aluminum pots and pans when cooking, and use deodorants that do not contain aluminum.

At present, however, there is no strong evidence to support the complete avoidance of aluminum products in everyday life.

Another toxin that has been investigated is the seed of a cycad plant (*Cycas circinalis*). This seed can cause a form of amyelotrophic lateral sclerosis (ALS, Lou Gehrig's disease), and Parkinson's disease. The cycad seed contains at least two poisonous neurotoxic agents. The plant is found in the Western Pacific islands of Guam, Rota, West New Guinea, and Japan, where people who consume it develop intellectual changes very similar to those seen in Alzheimer's disease.

It is also possible that an infectious agent is involved in Alzheimer's disease. No one has been able to identify a virus, and no aging animal model has been found so that the disease can be studied in the laboratory, although interesting similarities in brain cellular changes have been described in aged polar bears. It is too early to tell how helpful this will be.

14

MEDICAL TREATMENTS

The medical treatment of Alzheimer's disease is based on theory. At this point, no drug treatment is available to cure the disease. The decision to try a medication for the treatment of Alzheimer's disease should be made by the physician based on the wishes of the Alzheimer's sufferer as well as the medical history. As a rule, individuals in moderate to advanced stages of the disease or in poor general health are not accepted in experimental research drug trials. These individuals would probably not benefit from treatment because too much brain damage has occurred and the damage is irreversible. However, there are several avenues of research that may lead to clinical improvement in the initial stages of Alzheimer's disease.

Very early, research showed that the memory function of the brain cells, or neurons, requires *neurotransmitters*. These are chemicals that allow communication between the neurons. One of the essential neurotransmitters for memory function is acetylcholine (ACh). It is stored in the neurons until needed and is then released by the cells to be picked up by receptors or other brain cells. Acetylcholine is a product of choline, a component of lecithin, which we know as a dietary constituent of food and which can be purchased in most health food stores. Choline is converted into acetylcholine by the enzyme choline acetyltransferase (CAT). This enzyme is counteracted by acetylcholinesterase which destroys ACh, to achieve a stable balance.

In Alzheimer's disease, however, the level of acetylcholine is markedly decreased because the amount of the available enzyme choline acetyltransferase is reduced. Therefore, early attempts to treat Alzheimer's disease included increasing the consumption of lecithin or using compounds that slow the natural breakdown of acetylcholine in the brain by acetylcholinesterase, thereby increasing the life span and availability of acetylcholine. These experiments, tried on animals, such as rats, were fairly successful.

Unfortunately, the same success has not been achieved in humans. Perhaps this is because the brain cells themselves are damaged and cannot respond to acetylcholine or because many other transmitters are affected. Nonetheless, work continues with the development of agents that work against acetylcholinesterase, such as tetrahydroaminoacridine (THA, tacrine, or Cognex®). Very recently, a trial of THA offered some hope, but the drug was put on hold by the U.S. Food and Drug Administration (FDA) for larger use in the community because of unacceptable side effects of liver toxicity. It has now been approved for therapeutic trials in closely supervised settings, such as geriatric centers in the hospital. Further efforts in this direction should be promising.

Hydergine®

Hydergine® is probably the most frequently prescribed drug for the treatment of Alzheimer's disease. This drug is definitely not a cure for Alzheimer's disease. Nobody knows exactly how it works, but it appears to provide mild improvement in cognition and in mood. This may be due to an improvement in cerebral blood flow through opening of the vessels. The drug appears to be benign and may be worth a try, although there is conflicting information on its safety. It has been available in Europe for at least 25 years, but it only became approved by the FDA for use in dementia patients in the United States in 1984.

The usual dose is three milligrams per day, at a cost of $1 per tablet on average, or $90 per month. Some physicians recommend a double daily dose of six milligrams. A generic equivalent is available at a monthly cost of $6.24, but no cross-study is available. Recently, a study reported that

40

Hydergine® may actually provoke confusion and worsen memory. You may want to discuss this further with the physician.

Nootropics

These agents have been used mostly in Europe as "metabolic enhancers." Their goal is to make the existing brain cells work to their maximum potential without affecting blood flow and without serious side effects.

The most commonly used nootropic is piracetam, which has been used alone or in combination with choline.

Unfortunately, it has not been proved that the nootropics can ameliorate the cognitive decline of Alzheimer's disease. Researchers continue to investigate this interesting group of drugs.

Other Agents

There have been many other approaches to the treatment of Alzheimer's disease, which have been unsuccessful thus far. For your information, we mention the following:

Hyperbaric oxygen. Attempts to increase brain oxygenation by forcing oxygen using high-pressure chambers have been abandoned because of the lack of positive results.

Chelation therapy is a chemical process that attempts to clean the body by creating soluble complexes by adding metals or minerals. The theory is that the new substance is harmless because it cannot be used in this form by the body, but the procedure is dangerous, with serious risks to the heart, kidneys, and gastric system. It is also costly and of no proven benefit in Alzheimer's disease.

Narcotic antagonists. Naloxone may help to release more acetylcholine from the remaining functioning neurons in the brain. Trials have been done but without significant success.

Calcium channel blockers. Recent interest has been raised by the use of calcium channel blockers, such as Nimotop®. This medication affects the function of all cells, which depend on the availability of calcium. Theoretically, blocking the channels that permit calcium to enter and leave the cell may improve overall cellular performance. More research needs to be performed on this subject.

Eldepryl® **(selegiline)** is used in Parkinson's disease, another progressive neurological illness. Because some Alzheimer's victims seem to have neurotransmitter problems similar to those found in Parkinson's patients, trials have been done in Alzheimer's patients, using Eldepryl®. Results have been unconvincing thus far. In general, treated individuals appeared to be more sociable.

In summary, although many therapies are being investigated, none have managed to show a clear improvement of memory loss thus far. It is possible that the treatment of Alzheimer's disease will consist of a combination of drugs, each achieving a positive effect on a different affected neurotransmitter. Potentially all Alzheimer's victims may benefit from these and other drugs to be developed, but it is expected that the greater improvement will be seen in individuals with early to moderately advanced stages of dementia, because some of the brain cells remain intact. Unfortunately, in the early stage, individuals are generally physically healthy and it is very important to avoid dangerous or uncomfortable side effects. Discuss therapeutic options with the physician.

15

LIVING WITH AN ALZHEIMER'S SUFFERER

Living with a victim of Alzheimer's disease can be a very trying experience. Not all Alzheimer's victims progress at the same pace and exhibit the same behavioral problems, but many burden family caregivers with real concerns.

Early on, the first signs of memory failure may trigger irritation, frustration, and fear. Often, the individual is reprimanded by the spouse and told to pay attention or to be more reliable. The routine established over many years of life together has been disrupted. The individual with Alzheimer's no longer handles the everyday responsibilities he had carried for so many years: the garbage is not taken out every night, the mail is not picked up, and the dishes are no longer put away.

Tensions grow at home and in the family circle. At this point, the spouse is torn between denying the reality, attributing the observed memory loss to a passing illness or temporary stress, and recognizing the true problem by seeking medical help.

The first medical consultation for memory loss is a frightening experience for both victim and caregiver; the spouse usually knows what he or she is going to hear but still hopes for another answer.

As the disease progresses and the reality settles in, the spouse or responsible caregiver becomes burdened with all the decisions of efficiently running the household. What was a shared experience is now a heavy and lonely responsibility. At this stage, the caregiver often looks for help in the family. Siblings and children may be too busy with their own lives to extend themselves and accept sharing the task. Besides, they may be frightened themselves by the realization that mother or father is now aging and sick. Feelings of injustice, anger, and exhaustion begin to appear.

Finally, when the individual becomes physically dependent on the caregiver for most activities and demands practically nonstop attention, guilt often adds another emotional pressure. The slow progression of the disease sometimes leads to a death wish that the Alzheimer's patient would die soon, which is difficult to suppress, and "chronic grieving" is described by many caregivers.

The individual now follows the caregiver wherever he or she goes, from the bedroom to the bathroom, not allowing a single minute of peace or privacy. Often even sleep is disrupted.

Many studies have examined the stress level and burden of caregivers. It is generally recognized that at least one-third of Alzheimer's caregivers have some degree of emotional symptoms and physical problems.

It is important to remember that this emotional distress is perfectly normal and expected. Open discussions with the physician or other health care practitioner is an excellent way to recognize the existence of the mental turmoil and to take the first steps in resolving it. These steps may include professional counseling and joining support groups through the Alzheimer's Association, for instance. The Alzheimer's Association now has over 200 chapters throughout the United States. Their central number is 800-272-3900 (in Illinois, 800-572-6037). Participation is free of charge.

Also, some caregivers actually enjoy the new role of responsibility. They like to be in charge! Maybe these are people who have always been very nurturing and interested in providing hands-on care to other persons. Maybe these are people with a different motivation: they are trying to fill a void in their personal lives by taking on this new responsibility which might build up their self-esteem. Some children of Alzheimer's victims find this opportunity an excellent way to solve a personal conflict: a middle-aged single person will be devoted to caring for an Alzheimer's victim, justifying noninvolvement in a marital relationship and resolving loneliness. Being needed is nice!

In the meanwhile, several "tricks" can be used to make life more bearable:

1. Plan a scheduled respite time when you can treat yourself to a fun activity—maybe lunch with a friend, going to the movies, a walk in the park, an hour of window-shopping, or a game of golf or tennis. Arrange to hire a responsible person to take over at least once a week. This person may be a very good friend of yours, a student, or a volunteer from your religious affiliation (see Key 39).
2. Know your charge! Most individuals with Alzheimer's ask repeatedly for the same thing. Have the extra set of keys, eyeglasses, or papers ready to produce at any time of the day or night.
3. Keep cookies and finger foods handy; these are priceless during periods of agitation!
4. Give the Alzheimer's victim plenty of exercise, preferably outdoors. A brisk walk is good for both of you and helps you to sleep better at night.
5. Learn to "read" the individual with Alzheimer's. Certain situations always bother these individuals and trigger agitation. For example, many Alzheimer's victims react very negatively to the metallic sound of a doorbell. Consider changing the sound by purchasing a musical system. Certain television shows may be seen as a threat to an Alzheimer's victim. Avoid these shows, or lower the sound drastically.
6. If the individual suddenly appears much more agitated than normal, check for a physical cause: skin irritation, rash, constipation, or any kind of physical pain may be the reason for the agitation.
7. Use very graphic signs; a large "Stop, Do Not Enter" at the front door or your bedroom door may discourage wandering for awhile.

16

REALITY ORIENTATION

Reality orientation is a therapeutic approach geared at improving, through stimulations by sight, touch, and smell, understanding of the daily realities of life, such as the date, the time, the weather, special events, or holidays.

Many tools, including large-print calendars, clocks, posters, and holiday decorations, can be helpful and should be encouraged, particularly in the early to moderate stages of the disease. Often helpful are large pictures of family members, children, and grandchildren displayed on the refrigerator. A good idea is to write the names of these people in large print under the photographs.

However, there is a growing body of evidence that repeated "reality orientation sessions" in which the Alzheimer's victim is asked to formally rehearse the date or the weather are not helpful. In fact, this effort can be counterproductive, demeaning, and frustrating.

Reality orientation should be used gently in the course of normal conversation. For instance, rather than sitting down and stating, "We are now going to review today's date and schedule," casually mention, "Well, today is already the 20th of June, we are really moving into summer." Try to invite a natural response with a following question, such as, "Do you think this summer will be hot?"

One of the questions most often asked in a family counseling session is what to do when the Alzheimer's victim repeats exactly the same question.

• Do not point out that the individual is repeating himself. It is humiliating for him and contributes to increasing your sense of frustration.

- Gently repeat the same answer you gave last time. Remember, the individual is *not* doing this to upset you: she is sick.
- If the question becomes too repetitive, change the setting by distracting the individual with something new; take him for a walk, offer some food, or talk about something else.

Another frequent question is, "What do I do when she insists on telling me something wrong, such as repeating that a grandchild who lives out of town came to visit this morning?" As a rule, if there is no harm in it, let it be. Reality orientation in this context is not helpful. If the individual is sure that a pleasant event took place, so much the better. On the other hand, if the individual believes that something dreadful happened, then reassurance and sometimes distraction can do the trick. Paranoid feelings and hallucinations should be reported to the physician.

17

HOME SAFETY

As you learn to live with an individual with Alzheimer's disease, your primary concern becomes safety. As the disease progresses, individuals develop a tendency to fall because their gait becomes unstable. In addition, their impaired judgment does not allow them to protect themselves from daily hazards.

There are three dangerous areas in your home: the kitchen, the bathroom, and the exits (doors, windows, and balconies).

Kitchen

Most of us have forgotten a boiling pot on the stove. With the Alzheimer's victim, this becomes a daily experience, which can be particularly dangerous if the stove functions on gas rather than electricity. You should equip your stove with childproof locks. You can find these either in a store that sells children's furniture or in a major kitchen appliance store.

Bathroom

Bathrooms can become very slippery when water is spilled on the floor. Many dangerous falls occur in the bathroom. In addition, Alzheimer's victims may forget to turn off the water and cause floods. Do not use area rugs that can slip.

Another dangerous problem is the hot water. You can adjust the temperature of the hot water system to prevent a burn should the Alzheimer's victim get into a scalding hot bath or shower unattended.

Exits

Wandering out of the house may be extremely dangerous for Alzheimer's sufferers. In addition to the obvious dangers of traffic and possible muggings, the Alzheimer's victim may forget how to return home. The Alzheimer's Association offers a wide range of systems to tag patients (including clothing tags and identification bracelets) that are mandatory for the safety of these patients. You can also find identification bracelets in the local pharmacy or supermarket. The first step, however, is to ensure that the door is safely locked and that you will be notified if the door is opened. An alarm system, a bell, or a loud chime can alert you in the middle of the night that the Alzheimer's victim is trying to get out of the house.

A new lock with a special combination or a system that is difficult to open can give you peace of mind while you sleep. Remember, however, that this lock must be easy to open in case of fire. Under no circumstances leave the individual alone and unassisted in a locked home; this would be condemning him or her to death should a fire occur in your absence.

Check your windows. Many individuals with Alzheimer's, feeling physically fit, try to escape out of a window! Once again, children's furniture stores can help you in providing security devices.

Do not try to pile heavy furniture, such as sofas or tables, in front of exit doors. For one thing, they might not deter a strong individual from attempting to exit. Also, should there be an emergency in the middle of the night, you might find yourself trapped!

If despite all your precautions the individual wanders off, keep calm. Call the police immediately (911 if it is available in your area), and provide them with a recent photograph of your loved one. Try to add a good description of the clothes he or she was wearing when last seen. The police are very familiar with such situations and very understanding. Wait at home for phone calls. Not infrequently, the individual will have wandered off on a familiar path to a neighbor's home or a child's or even to his or her former office. Chances are that you will soon receive a reassuring call.

You may want to use a checklist to ensure the safety of your home, or your children's home if you visit frequently. Does your spouse leave the door unlocked, the oven on, or the water running? This will help you focus on possible hazards. Make sure you have the local poison control number and doctor's number available by the telephone.

	Area to Check	What to Do
Entrance door(s)	Steps	Install a handrail.
	Lock	Place an inside lock to be used with a key, to avoid wandering.
Windows		Install guardlocks.
Stairs	Steps and light	Keep stairs free of objects that could cause a fall. Do not wax stairs. Install good lighting.
Bathroom	Medication cabinet	Remove all toxic chemicals to a separate locked unit. Discard what you no longer need. Consider using childproof containers for your own medications.
	Toilet	Install a grab bar.
	Bathtub	Avoid using a floor mat. Avoid
	Sink	electrical appliances. Install a vanity around the sink.
Kitchen	Stove and oven	Consider a cutoff switch for the stove or childproof guards for switches.
General	Electrical cords and outlets	Replace frayed cords. Fasten cords along the walls.
	Green plants Dieffenbachia Caladium Poinsettia Philodendron Ivy Lily of the valley Rhododendron Hydrangea Laurel Yew Elephant ears	Avoid buying these poisonous plants. If you have them already, place them out of reach.
	Area rugs	Remove them, or tack them down.

18

WHEN AND HOW TO STOP DRIVING A CAR

One of the biggest problems with the daily management of individuals with Alzheimer's disease is the discrepancy between their mental and physical abilities. They cannot remember things, but they walk and behave like nondemented people. For this reason, many feel that they are perfectly capable of driving the car as they have for so many years.

In the early stages of the illness, when only memory is affected and judgment is intact, there is no reason to stop the individual from driving. However, you or another responsible caregiver must go along so that the Alzheimer's victim does not become lost. This may mean that you keep the keys to the car because the individual with Alzheimer's will not remember to ask you to come along.

As the disease progresses and judgment becomes impaired, it becomes dangerous to allow Alzheimer's victims to drive. Life and death decisions must be made in a fraction of a second, before you have a chance to interject and order the individual to turn or brake to avoid a child, an animal, or another car. It is safer at this point to have the person give up driving. Unfortunately, the burden is on your shoulders as the responsible caregiver. Motor vehicle departments are not equipped to test mental function and therefore do not assist you in this process.

The following approach is usually helpful:

- Enroll the help of the physician. Ask him or her whether the Alzheimer's victim can still drive. If the answer is no, have the doctor explain, in your presence, the dangers of continuing to drive. It might be helpful to get from your physician a prescription note with the following words: "Do Not

Drive." You can tape the prescription on the inside of the front door.

- Hide the keys.
- Park the car out of the individual's sight. You might be able to leave the car on the street or in a friendly neighbor's driveway.
- If you can drive, insist on driving yourself rather than allowing the Alzheimer's victim to drive. You can give the following reasons:

   The doctor says that you should not drive.

   I feel like driving today.

   You have done so much today—let me do something.

   I know the way; you can rest now and enjoy yourself later.
- If you do not drive, sell the car. This is one less hassle for you to deal with. Explore with a local taxi company the costs of regular weekly or biweekly trips to the supermarket, the movie theater, or the hairstylist. Taxi companies often schedule shared rides at convenient times for affordable rates.
- Check the local *Pennysaver* or local newspaper; retired people sometimes offer their services as drivers or to run errands.
- Call the supermarket and pharmacy; they may deliver goods for a minimal charge.
- Look into public transportation systems and at your senior citizen center for organized trips. You can discover a world out there even without a car!

19

WHEN TO RETIRE

Retire before you are asked to do so!

If you or your loved one has been diagnosed as having Alzheimer's disease, the time to start planning retirement is now. Alzheimer's is a slowly progressive disease. Once the physician has made the diagnosis, memory troubles increase and eventually judgment is impaired. These dysfunctions obviously interfere with efficient work production, and the burden of catching up and correcting mistakes falls on colleagues. This leads only to resentment and upset in the workplace.

A transition period should be implemented, during which active projects can be transferred to other responsible workers, papers completed, and arrangements made for hiring or promoting colleagues.

In addition, many time-consuming legal and financial matters need to be settled on the home front. These matters take time away from work hours and should be given priority. Remember, very few insurance companies provide any kind of coverage for the long-term care of chronic illnesses, or for nursing homes. Medicare, the federal health care program for all citizens over the age of 65, *does not cover* any of these costs unless the Alzheimer's patient has just been hospitalized and requires skilled nursing care that can only be rendered in a skilled nursing home and only for a limited period of time. You should now look into your pension plan and benefits and investigate the private long-term insurance companies. Some large companies offer Employee Assistance programs which are designed to help with caregiving responsibilities.

Be ready for a difficult period that may bring depression. Consider short-term psychotherapy for both you and your loved ones to help with the adjustment to a new life-style.

20

SOCIAL ACTIVITIES AND HOBBIES

There is no reason not to encourage the continuation of social activities and hobbies or perhaps start new ones. The only drawback is often the individual's attitude. People suffering from Alzheimer's disease tend to isolate themselves, perhaps out of embarrassment or anxiety in front of friends. They realize they are not performing as well as they used to, and they would rather not demonstrate this loss publicly. Keeping in mind this shyness, the spouse or other caregiver should make every effort to encourage continued socialization.

Sports

If the individual enjoys sports, such as tennis, golf, or swimming, these activities should be continued because Alzheimer's victims usually remain physically healthy and continue to perform well until much later in the course of the disease. Make sure that there is always someone with the individual to oversee the activity and avoid errors in judgment. You don't want the individual to be lost on the golf course or swim out to sea. Be sensitive to the feelings of the sport partner. An old tennis partner may no longer want to play with your spouse, who now shows signs of Alzheimer's disease. In this respect, individual sports are often a better choice.

Music

The "music center" in the brain is generally not affected during the early and middle stages of the Alzheimer's process. Famous musicians suffering from Alzheimer's disease can still perform an entire symphony without mistakes! Songs and melodies remain in our minds. Sing-alongs, operettas, and other musical productions can be great activities for the Alzheimer's victim.

Games

Games requiring memory skills and concentration become frustrating. In our experience, card games should be limited to close family members and friends, who will play along rather than compete. For the same reason, young children who cannot yet understand their grandparent's condition should not be encouraged to play these kinds of games because they may verbalize their disappointment when Grandpa doesn't remember which card to choose, and this may provoke feelings of hurt and worthlessness.

Hobbies

Because individuals with Alzheimer's tend to enjoy one-on-one activities, new hobbies should be suggested. Among those that we have found most helpful are gardening, drawing, painting, collage, pottery, and other therapeutic activities conducive to peaceful and pleasant times. Most towns have an arts and crafts store where inexpensive materials can be purchased. Creativity and imagination are the keys.

Household Activities

Many of the individuals with Alzheimer's who are our patients have been set up in homemaking routines. It is very reassuring and soothing for them to continue with the tasks of daily routine even when the purpose of these tasks is lost. For instance, one individual with very advanced Alzheimer's found peace in folding and unfolding the same sheet over and over again. In fact, her daughter noted that this newly found activity curbed the victim's incessant pacing.

Allowing individuals to help with household tasks, such as drying the dishes, may also provide a sense of usefulness and self-esteem.

Baby-sitting

A major area of concern is of course baby-sitting. Young children should not be left to the care of a grandparent with Alzheimer's who has memory and judgment impairment. Alzheimer's victims can be left with a responsible teenager, however, provided you have a clear understanding with the young adult of who is watching whom.

21

WHAT TO TELL COLLEAGUES AND FRIENDS

Avoiding the truth or trying to cover up for the individual with Alzheimer's disease creates an enormous and stressful burden on you. Friends tend to pull away and not socialize because they can no longer relate well to you or freely discuss their concerns about your sick spouse. They are reacting to subtle changes in the individual's behavior: perhaps a sense of hostility in the conversation, a feeling of depression, or more apathy in their social demeanor.

Your best approach is the honest truth. Be sure that if you have noticed changes, so have they! You need not provide comprehensive details on the extent of the difficulties or the medical workup you have undergone. However, a general statement indicating that you are aware of the memory trouble and that you are taking the appropriate steps will clear the air.

You may want to say, "We have all been concerned about Jack's memory. We took him to a specialist, who thinks it is probably Alzheimer's disease."

In general, such a statement produces a reaction of understanding and compassion that will be helpful to you and to your loved one. Everyone has heard of Alzheimer's disease, and many have encountered Alzheimer's victims among family or friends. Alzheimer's disease is no longer perceived as a strange psychiatric illness in which people lose their minds.

By discussing the problem openly with your friends, you allow them to partake, if they wish, in the care of the Alzheimer's victim. People usually enjoy sharing their own problems and may suggest helpful and constructive approaches to deal with your problem. Often, they very willingly readjust their expectations of a game partner, for example. A bridge game becomes less competitive and more of a social gathering. The bridge partner might welcome a new role, that of a caring and compassionate person extending the hand of friendship. A work colleague may be quite relieved to find out that you are indeed aware of the problem. This common knowledge of the situation enables both of you to make realistic plans for settling tasks at work, reorganizing, reassigning responsibilities, and planning retirement. A frank discussion with your spouse's supervisor or with the Human Resources department of the company should include a review of disability benefits to which he or she may be entitled, depending on the company's health care benefit package. (See the Appendix for Additional Reading.)

22

WHAT TO TELL CHILDREN AND GRANDCHILDREN

If someone in your family suffers from Alzheimer's disease, explain the issue to the youngsters who may meet the person at the next family gathering.

Once again, the best approach with children and grandchildren is the truth: "Grandma has a problem with her memory; she cannot always remember things well."

You may want to propose a method in dealing with the problem: "If Grandpa repeats something he told you a few minutes ago, please don't hurt his feelings by telling him he is repeating himself. Just listen to it again; it will make him feel good."

Most children are pleased to participate in the "therapeutic" handling of the patient and feel privileged to be part of the family team. However, we should also remember that they are children and may become impatient or frustrated. They should not be blamed or made to feel guilty or shameful for such feelings. A possible suggestion is: "If you get frustrated, just excuse yourself and go to another room. It's okay to get upset sometimes."

Be receptive to children's questions. Sit down with them when you know you will have some quiet time to listen patiently to them without interruption. Bedtime is best. They are likely to raise key issues, depending on their age, level of maturity, and concern. For instance, a child might ask, "Does this mean Grandma is going to die soon?" The answer, of course, is "No, her heart is good and strong and we can continue to have many happy days together." Another question might be, "If Grandpa kisses me, will I catch this disease, too?" Reassure the child by saying that this is not a "catching" illness like a cold or chicken pox. This is an illness that affects some people when they get very, very old. Some children then follow this statement by asking, "Will I ever get it?" Here again, the answer is, "Probably not, but anyway, even if you ever do, it will be in a long, long time and the doctors may well have a cure for it then."

Finally, many children voice the concern we all have: "Will it get worse?" The answer is yes, but very slowly and progressively. The important thing for all of us is to truly enjoy the present and make the most out of it.

Older children and teenagers often express their embarrassment at having friends call them on the telephone only to be greeted by a demented grandfather, or visiting them at home while Grandma carries on. It is essential to develop a working partnership with your teenager in which mutual privacy becomes a golden rule. Enroll his or her help in finding a good respite program in the community and perhaps assisting you in transporting the Alzheimer's victim to the center on a prearranged schedule. Your teenager is then free to entertain friends at home while Grandma or Grandpa is at the center.

Several books for children have recently been published on the topic of Alzheimer's disease. (See the Appendix for Additional Reading.)

23

PET THERAPY

One of the best treatment modalities for individuals with Alzheimer's disease is pet therapy. A gentle, well-selected animal never provokes the frustration that the company of humans may. Pets do not ask questions that challenge the memory, and they never snap back if you repeat yourself. Any animal can represent a good distraction for Alzheimer's victims, but we prefer dogs because they can play an important role in general safety besides offering entertainment and companionship.

Several breeds are recommended. Labrador retrievers are smart, gentle, and usually well-behaved in the home setting. They are easy to groom and do not require an extraordinary amount of attention. English springer spaniels are joyful and cheerful companions. Outgoing, friendly, and sometimes silly, they require more physical activity. German shepherds are excellent watchdogs but need good obedience training. The smaller breeds, such as miniature poodles, schnauzers, and terriers, tend to be easily distracted and noisy and can be dangerous to safety because elderly people can trip on them.

Other pets, such as cats, rabbits, and fish, may be helpful if dogs cannot be kept in the apartment setting. Cats should be declawed or clipped regularly to reduce damage to people and furniture.

Obviously, the health care of the animal becomes an additional burden for the caregiver. However, the overall benefits of this nondemanding companionship are well worth the investment.

An inexpensive way to adopt an animal is to visit your local animal shelter. Ask why the animal was brought to the shelter. Did it bite anyone? Was it barking too much? Was it difficult to housebreak? Did the owners simply change their minds? An intelligent supervisor will respond honestly to your questions to avoid having the animal returned to the shelter one more time after you find out the real problem. Be aware that most animal shelters will provide you with a special package for a series of vaccinations against pet illnesses, a treatment against worms (a common ailment of dogs), and neutering or spaying intervention. Unless you are set on raising young puppies, it is an excellent idea to have the animal neutered before taking it home. It will be much more manageable in the long run. When you choose the animal, select one that comes readily to you, wags its tail, and appears content. Stay away from a lethargic, uninterested puppy. Don't bother to visit the shelter until you have pretty much made up your mind to adopt; these animals have a great talent to become irresistible and steal your heart!

You may want to check your local newspaper for animals available for adoption. Be sure that you check the return policy before getting an animal. You should be able to bring it back to its previous owner within at least a week if unforeseen problems occur.

Remember, you will continue to be responsible for the pet after the Alzheimer's victim dies, or is admitted to a nursing home. You should feel comfortable in assuming the long-term care and responsibilities of this animal.

24

TRAVELING

Travel only if you must!

Traveling can be very pleasant but can also cause unnecessary anxiety. In our experience, most individuals with Alzheimer's disease do not enjoy leaving their familiar surroundings. Indeed, they prefer to receive visitors at home rather than travel to "unknown" settings.

If traveling must be imposed, try to select dates and times that will not be too busy. An airport during a holiday season has a frantic pace. For a demented individual, this can be a most distressing experience. Harried personnel are unable to provide the extra help and individualized attention required. Ask the travel agent for the best routes and schedules. Midmorning flights Monday through Thursday are usually best.

Discuss with your physician the appropriate sedation to be used in an emergency. Short-term sedation is not very dangerous and can be of great help. It may be wise to try the medication at home once, to make sure that the individual doesn't have the opposite reaction—agitation. Also, the test may give you a good idea of how long this medication will take to start working and how long it will last. Types of medications used for sedation include Valium®, Ativan®, Haldol®, and Mellaril®.

When you travel, always have a change of clothes ready and plenty of snacks. Carry towelettes and tissues in case of spills.

Consider a companion for the trip, either a family member or a paid home health attendant. This takes a large burden from your shoulders if you must wait on line for ticketing or for luggage while the Alzheimer's victim becomes agitated.

Exercise extra caution in public places; an individual suffering from Alzheimer's disease can easily wander away during a short moment of inattention.

If you have a companion, clarify from the beginning what you will pay for and what expenses the companion can expect to bear. Many people are anxious to travel to warmer climates during the winter and would be willing to help you out in exchange for a free airline ticket. Spell out the duration of the trip and the specific expected duties: "I will pick you up at 8 A.M. on Friday at your house and leave you at the Miami Airport upon our arrival at 2 P.M. I expect you to stay with Marvin at all times and accompany him to the toilet if he needs to go."

Driving your own car for shorter trips gives you more flexibility. Unfortunately, it is difficult to concentrate on the road while keeping the Alzheimer's victim comfortable and quiet. Again, you will be better off leaving in the morning and planning a rest stop every two to three hours.

Do not plan any event immediately following your arrival. It is best for you to settle into the hotel or the vacation home before introducing the additional stress of new faces, family members, friends, or neighbors.

Make sure when you arrive in your new setting that you check it for adequate safety (see Key 17). You may want to bring along safety chains and locks.

Overall, be sure that the trip will be worthwhile for you as well as for your loved one, before you embark on it!

25

AT THE RESTAURANT

If you have been used to eating in restaurants, there is no reason to change this habit now. You may want to select a different type of establishment, however. A formal dining place with elaborate service may produce a negative reaction in an impatient Alzheimer's sufferer, who is anxious to get up and walk around.

In general, these individuals do well in diners that offer fast, competent, and friendly service or in family restaurants with self-service buffets where customers can get up and walk without attracting attention.

Try to get to the restaurant early, between 5 and 6 P.M. You will avoid waiting on line, which can be disastrous. Once at the table, try to get a basket of bread as soon as possible. Remove all confusing utensils, salt and pepper shakers, and ashtrays if they seem to disturb the patient.

Suggest finger food, which is easy to reach and easy to handle. Chicken fingers, fresh vegetables, pieces of cheese, bread, and cake are wonderful and nutritious foods. Avoid soups, spaghetti, or complicated sandwiches; they are confusing and frustrating to Alzheimer's victims, who are unsure of what utensils to use and where to start. Do not allow fish with bones, fruits with small pits that can be swallowed (such as prunes and apricots), or hot dogs with skin that can make the individual choke. You may want to take along wet napkins or towelettes to clean the fingers.

You may need to rescue the poor waiter, as the Alzheimer's victim in your care keeps ordering the same food item over and over again. Try to go to a restaurant without waiters, such as a fast-food establishment. If you can't avoid it and a problem arises, you can always speak briefly to the server and make it clear that you will tip appropriately.

Find out immediately where the restrooms are, in case you need one urgently. If you choose a restaurant where the bathroom is on the ground level rather than downstairs in the basement, so much the better. Also be prepared to pay quickly using cash rather than credit cards and leave if your loved one shows signs of agitation. You may have an additional problem if the Alzheimer's sufferer was used to paying the bill. Often you see him reaching repeatedly for a credit card or wallet with mounting anxiety. Just repeat firmly, "Tonight, it's my treat." You may add, "If you want to leave the tip, why don't you leave a few dollars on the table." Make sure that the Alzheimer's victim in your care has the few dollars needed.

There is no reason to abstain from a moderate amount of alcohol. In fact, a little bit of wine may produce slight sedation, which might help on the return home. On the way out, avoid the large candy mints, which are easy to choke on.

26

SEX

Individuals with Alzheimer's disease are usually physically healthy. Most tend to continue their normal patterns of sexual activity. However, there is great variation in the normal sexual patterns of elderly couples, from daily intercourse to complete abstinence.

The intimate relationship sought by the individual should be continued as long as is comfortable for both partners. Remember that simple physical contact, caressing and holding, can be very reassuring and pleasing to both partners. There is no medical reason to abstain from sex in Alzheimer's disease. In fact, many individuals with Alzheimer's continue to be sexually active well into the advanced stages of the disease.

Some forms of dementia, primarily affecting the frontal lobes of the brain (that is, the area behind the forehead), can cause sexual hyperactivity as a result of decreased inhibition, which normally limits our sexual expressions to appropriate settings and circumstances according to learned social rules. Depending on the needs of the partner, this increased activity can be welcome, repulsive, or tolerable. If the partner is not willing to participate, the individual feels rejected and may react with outbursts of anger and agitation.

The spouse is often so angry that he or she becomes unable to participate in sexual intimacy. A short course of psychotherapy helps to clarify, accept, and resolve the sources of this anger. Better understanding of the prior sexual relationship of the couple and ongoing expectations are very helpful. In the advanced stages, the individual may no longer recognize the bed partner and refuse or reject sexual advances. This is often very difficult to accept for a devoted spouse who is now accused of being an impostor or a prostitute. In addition, there are often further complications, such as urinary frequency or urinary incontinence at night and sleeplessness. The spouse may be simply too exhausted to volunteer or even to participate in sexual activity.

If the pattern and frequency of sexual encounters become intolerable to the nondemented spouse, medications to sedate the victim are available. Discuss your needs as well as those of the Alzheimer's victim with the physician.

27

SLEEP AND CIRCADIAN RHYTHM

Sleep patterns change with normal aging. The infant and young child require up to 20 hours of sleep a day, but the young adult generally sleeps about 8 hours per day and the elderly adult functions on 5 to 6 hours per day, with perhaps a catnap in the afternoon. This normal daily (*circadian*) sleep-wake cycle is affected in Alzheimer's disease. Afflicted individuals often demonstrate reverse cycles with frequent periods of sleep during the day and awakening at night.

The transition period of the late afternoon, the *sundown period*, is particularly troublesome, marked by agitation, pacing, restlessness, and anxiety. Research studies on Alzheimer's victims during sleep have shown changes from normal aging patterns in the rapid eye movement observed during dream periods.

The lack of sleep at night creates an enormous burden for the already exhausted caregiver, and it is important that every effort be made to improve this situation.

Standard sleep hygiene rules for both Alzheimer's sufferers and caregivers include the following:

1. Do not use the bedroom when you are not planning to sleep. Do not stay in bed to read, eat, or watch television. The brain should be conditioned to associate bed with sleep only.
2. Do not eat a heavy meal or drink caffeine products for at least two hours before your sleep time.
3. Do not overheat the bedroom; maintain a cool temperature, around 68 to 70°F.
4. Do not encourage naps during the day.

5. Do not go to bed too early. Many elderly people get into bed at 7 P.M. and are surprised to find themselves awake in the early hours of the morning.
6. Encourage the Alzheimer's victim to get into nightclothes such as pajamas. Do not leave day clothes out, because the individual with Alzheimer's who wakes in the middle of the night may well attempt to get dressed.
7. Get plenty of exercise, preferably outdoors, during the day.

If these standard rules fail to help, the doctor can prescribe a sleeping pill or an antidepressant medication with a sedative effect, such as trazodone, to be taken at night. (See Key 34.) Sleeping pills are effective for short periods of time. Unfortunately, after awhile they lose their potency. Increased doses are then required, raising the possibility of addiction. Some sleeping medications have a long duration of action; others are very short acting, perhaps for only four to six hours. Long-acting medications are not advisable in elderly people because these persons have a slower metabolism and a different body composition. Drugs tend to stay in the system for a much longer period of time than in younger individuals. Be aware that sleeping pills have side effects, which include daytime drowsiness, worsening of memory and confusion, and increased risk of falls. The newer medications have fewer side effects, however, and can be of great help in the daily management of these individuals.

28

HYGIENE

As individuals progress to the moderately advanced stages of the disease, they forget when and how to wash themselves, brush their teeth, and comb their hair. You, as caregiver, must at first offer cues and then eventually total assistance. Do not expect the Alzheimer's victim to remember to brush his teeth. Do not get upset or angry when she forgets to do so.

Grooming

We suggest that you consider making a weekly appointment at the local hair salon for women and every month to six weeks for men. Choose a hairstyle that is easy to care for, and ask the stylist how best to comb the hair between appointments. Most stylists are delighted to offer advice.

If the individual with Alzheimer's is used to applying makeup, continue to purchase the cosmetics she likes—lipstick and blush for the cheeks, for instance. Most department stores carry a large selection of products. Bring along the lipstick she usually wears to the department store. The salesperson will be able to identify the correct shade with much greater ease than if you tried to describe it. Allow your spouse to apply the makeup; lead her to a mirror and praise her. Later you can correct any excess.

Bathing

Bathing becomes a major problem. Many individuals with Alzheimer's refuse to wash and bathe. They may express a fear of entering the tub or shower. Purchase a shower or tub bench at a surgical supply store, which allows the individual to sit comfortably while washing. Install a shower curtain rather than a glass shower door; this allows more flexibility. Also, have a grab bar installed in the tub or shower area. Some people do not like water on their faces. A hand-held shower nozzle is a good solution. If the individual expresses discomfort at getting undressed in front of you, use towels to cover him or her and temporarily uncover only the area to be washed.

Remember that elderly people do not require daily bathing. The skin is dry and too much soap or washing can create irritation. Unless the individual is incontinent of urine and feces and has a strong body odor, you can get by with a weekly bath, as long as you wash the face, underarms, and groin area at least once a day.

Overall, make sure that you don't hurt yourself while assisting in the bath. Bathrooms are slippery areas. If you try to assist an agitated individual on a wet bathroom floor, you may fall. Consider hiring an experienced home health care person for thorough bathing once a week. The number of the local health care agency can be found in the Yellow Pages under Nurses.

Oral Health Care

The individual with Alzheimer's often needs assistance with oral health care whether or not he or she has dentures.

Oral hygiene is important to prevent the probability of decay of the existing teeth and serious infections. One of the major goals of the health practitioner is to maintain a painless and peaceful quality of life, and this includes avoiding toothaches and sore gums!

Care of Teeth and Gums

Teeth should be brushed twice a day at a minimum, in the morning and at night before bed. However, the techniques for brushing teeth in Alzheimer's victims can be modified to achieve efficient removal of large food debris and plaque without having the individual gag or choke on foaming toothpaste.

First, purchase a small toothbrush, which is much easier to manipulate and to remove from an agitated individual's mouth.

Be sure that the toothbrush is soft. With normal aging, gums recede, exposing the unprotected root of the tooth. Aggressive brushing with a hard toothbrush may damage the base of the tooth.

Second, you may want to forget about using toothpaste. A wet toothbrush is sufficient to remove large pieces of food on the teeth. The major benefit of toothpaste is the fluoride, which helps prevent decay. However, a toothpaste produces foam, which in turn should be rinsed and spat out. Most individuals with Alzheimer's are unable to spit out the paste on command. By foregoing the toothpaste, you avoid a regular battle of spitting versus swallowing.

Third, as long as you are not using toothpaste, you no longer require water, or even a sink. Therefore, brushing the individual's teeth can take place in a familiar, nonthreatening area, such as the kitchen or dining room. In fact, you might choose to place the individual in a comfortable armchair.

Fourth, in caring for individuals in advanced stages of the disease who are unable to brush their teeth unassisted, you may want to position yourself slightly behind, near the ear, to support the head against you while you proceed. With one hand, gently hold the lips apart while you brush with the other hand. When able, be sure to brush all the surfaces of the tooth, inside and out, not only the tops of the teeth. Always carefully rinse the toothbrush when you are done, and remember to change the toothbrush every three months.

Care of Dentures

In the United States, over 50 percent of elderly people are toothless to one degree or another. Many individuals with Alzheimer's remember how to handle dentures because they have done it for so many years, but you may need to learn to assist them eventually. Here are some helpful hints.

First, find out if the individual has a full denture (all the teeth are artificial) or a partial denture (some of the teeth are artificial and hook onto the individual's existing teeth). Some partial prostheses are quite difficult to remove, and you should have the dentist instruct you on proper techniques. A full upper denture should be removed by applying one finger above the rim on each side of the denture and firmly pulling downward. For lower complete dentures, one finger goes under the denture ridge and lifts upward. Why should you bother to insert the dentures? The individual will look better, feel better, eat better, and speak better. Perhaps even more importantly, because the individual looks more "together," he or she commands more respect from others. Why should you bother to take the dentures out at night? Because individuals who wear dentures at night have a higher incidence of fungal infections and sores. Dentures must be removed, cleaned thoroughly with a toothbrush, and kept in water. There is no need to add a product to the water unless the individual enjoys the taste.

Dentures are expensive. A full set of upper and lower dentures can cost $1500. Many individuals with Alzheimer's lose or break dentures. Replacing these dentures is costly, not reimbursed by Medicare, and very time consuming. A new pair of dentures, like a new pair of slippers, may take months to get used to. You can help avoid this with the following precautions.

- If the individual is used to removing his own dentures in the bathroom, always fill the sink with water and place a towel on the bottom of the sink to act as a cushion. A denture that falls into an empty sink can break.
- Have the dentist label the dentures with the individual's name. Should she ever be admitted to a hospital and the dentures misplaced, the chances of retrieving them will be much greater.
- Get in the habit of checking napkins and tissues before you throw them out. Many individuals take out the dentures during a meal if food is caught in them and wrap the food and the denture in a napkin.

- Use adhesive paste or powder only if the individual truly needs it, that is, if the dentures are loose. This decision should be left to an experienced dentist.

Finally, as a rule, plan a checkup with a good dentist every six months. The purpose of this checkup is to provide a thorough examination and cleaning of the oral cavity, whether or not there are teeth and an opportunity to screen for oral manifestations of *systemic disease* (affecting the body as a whole) or oral cancer, which is seen more frequently in elderly people.

*Acknowledgment: The authors express their gratitude to Sheryl Silverstein, D.M.D. for her expert and gracious assistance with the oral health care section.

29

SELECTING CLOTHES
AND DRESSING

Alzheimer's victims lose their judgment and can no longer select clothes that are appropriate for the weather, the season, and the function. In addition, they are fearful of change and want to continue wearing the clothes they have on rather than face the frustration of removing them and replacing them with unknown and difficult to find items.

You will need help. First, try to simplify things for yourself and for your loved one. Keep a small selection of useful, easy to put on, and *washable* (that is, machine washable; check the inside label) clothes in the closet. You may want to consider purchasing a basic functional wardrobe. We suggest, for *men*, one or two jogging suits with elastic waistbands, one or two pairs of trousers, two polo shirts, two dress shirts, and one blazer; for *women*, pants or a jogging suit if she appears comfortable in it, and two dresses, preferably with front buttons or zippers, which make it easy to open and close. Make sure that the dress is large enough to fit comfortably around the waist, particularly if she must wear diapers.

Underwear should be all cotton. A brassiere should fit comfortably without leaving pressure marks on the shoulders. If you have never purchased a bra before, ask a salesperson to help you. The size depends on the width measured under the breasts, usually 36 to 40 inches. The size of the cup goes from A to D for very large breasts. Therefore, you might be looking for a 36B for an average person or a 38D if the woman has larger breasts. A slip is generally not required because it complicates use of the toilet and undressing. Pantyhose can be purchased in supermarkets, although it may be cumbersome to put on. To select them, follow the guidelines on the back of the package according to height and weight. Avoid knee-high stockings, which may create compression in the calf area.

Check the shoes; they should fit comfortably and leave no pressure marks on the feet. Avoid shoelaces, which may become untied. A low heel is always preferable. Slip-on sneakers are very convenient.

To dress the individual with Alzheimer's, display the selected clothing on the bed and encourage the individual to get dressed. You may want to dress yourself at the same time, offering visual cues. If the individual doesn't respond, then offer your assistance. In addition to clothing, consider providing a handbag for women with a few items such as tissue, wallet with some change, and pictures. A man may like to have a pen or a credit card wallet. Sometimes old credit cards may help quiet the Alzheimer's person.

Communicate with your loved one by explaining in a matter-of-fact manner what you are doing: "John, here is your shirt, let's put your arm in the sleeve; there; here you are; now, let's button the shirt." Do not offer open-ended questions, such as "What would you like to wear today?" This provokes anxiety because the individual has no idea of what to wear. If you want to give a choice, select two items, and state, "Here are your two shirts; do you prefer the blue one or the red one?" Should John hesitate, don't push him to make a decision. Take one of the shirts, and begin to dress him while saying "That blue one will suit you very well." Do not forget at night to help him select appropriate and comfortable nightclothes. These serve as a visual cue that the time has come to go to bed.

30

AGITATION

Agitation is an emotional state of inner turmoil that manifests itself by physical motions, such as pacing and handwringing. In extreme cases, agitated individuals may become dangerous to themselves and others, especially when consistently provoked. By and large, however, the majority of individuals suffering from Alzheimer's do not represent any danger to their loved ones.

Agitation is rarely seen in the early stages unless the individual has had a lifelong tendency to worry. With these individuals, the perception that there is memory loss—in other words, that there is something wrong—creates a feeling of anxiety and upset. Not finding one's keys or one's eyeglasses can promote such distress that the individual loses sleep.

Agitation in these individuals often accompanies a depressed mood. The individual begins to pace back and forth with a worried look on her face. This affects everyone she comes in contact with, in particular her spouse. The spouse then becomes annoyed. His reaction triggers further agitation with verbal altercation.

By closely observing the individual, you may be able to identify those factors that trigger agitation. One of our patients would wake up regularly in the middle of the night looking for his tax documents. Eventually, his wife photocopied the documents and left a copy in her nightstand, which she would retrieve whenever he searched for them.

Many individuals become preoccupied and agitated about money, checking their wallets incessantly. As a rule, it is better to allow them their routine rather than confront them with the uselessness of this particular behavior.

Avoiding the onset of agitation is ideal but not always possible. Once the individual becomes agitated, stay calm. Make an effort to speak softly and slowly. Check that there is no physical discomfort caused by pain, hunger, thirst, or wet underpants. The individual may respond to one-on-one reassurance, to a food treat, or merely to being given a chance to express his or her feelings.

Physical exercise, as recommended by the doctor, may produce a decrease in the agitation and induce a beneficial fatigue. Music is sometimes helpful. Some of our caregivers attempt to distract agitated Alzheimer's victims by offering a different stimulus as a distraction. A dresser with several drawers reserved for the exclusive use of the Alzheimer's victim enables him or her to rummage to their heart's content.

Persistent agitation may signal the need for antidepressants, such as nortriptyline, with frequent visits to a geriatrician or psychiatrist to monitor the medication and its side effects. Other medications that can be very useful in easing the symptoms of agitation are minor and major tranquilizers. (See Key 34.)

Going with the flow—not arguing with the individual even though you are right—is the way to go. Peace and tranquility in the home are more important than proving yourself correct!

In the later stages of the disease, agitation is commonly seen as the brain no longer functions normally. The individual is often incoherent, mumbling and repeating sounds without meaning. At this stage, medications may not work any longer and the individual may need to be transferred to a safe environment, such as an Alzheimer's unit in a nursing home. It is essential for the medical team to continuously monitor the individual for possible physical causes of discomfort that may be creating or increasing the level of agitation. Rarely must one use physical restraints, such as belts or vests, to hold down the individual. Be aware that any form of restraint is a serious medical act and requires your designated representative, that is, the responsible caregiver's consent.

31

PARANOIA

Paranoia is described by the American Psychiatric Association as "unwarranted suspiciousness and mistrust of people." This symptom was actually one of the many symptoms described in 1907 by Alzheimer. The woman portrayed in his original case report accused her husband of adultery. Many individuals with Alzheimer's may question a spouse's loyalty with pathological jealousy. For example, an Alzheimer's victim may tell his children that his 84-year-old arthritic and debilitated wife is having an affair with the young mailman.

The most frequent example of *paranoid ideation* (paranoid thought process) is the idea that someone is stealing. Alzheimer's victims can suspect people of stealing objects or money from them because they have misplaced things and cannot remember where to find them. Sometimes, the individual selects a specific person in the household as the "culprit," to the relief of the other family members. Extra sets of keys, frequent reminders of where they put an object (your bag is on the chair), and attaching eyeglasses around the neck with a decorative chain are helpful tricks. Obviously, one should not leave important papers or large sums of money with an Alzheimer's victim who is likely to misplace them.

Paranoid ideations usually appear in the early to middle stages of the illness. With progression and worsening of intellectual function, these individuals lose the ability to formulate paranoid thoughts. This is therefore a transient stage, which is important information for you as a caregiver. Paranoia can be very distressing for the family and home help, but it is essential to remember that this is part of Alzheimer's disease, not a personal accusation. Not all Alzheimer's victims develop paranoia. It seems that people who have had compulsive personalities are more likely to exhibit these symptoms.

As with agitation, certain individuals exhibited mistrust and suspicion of other people's motivations before ever developing memory loss. Unfortunately, the Alzheimer's victim with these preexisting traits becomes worse as he or she loses control and forgets learned social graces.

In any case, paranoia should prompt medical consultation to determine whether it should be treated with drugs. When paranoia appears it usually remains a prominent feature until treated. The individual is paranoid every day, all day. Toward the end of the disease, the individual is no longer able to organize his or her thoughts enough to express a paranoid concept, and medications may no longer be required.

It is not easy for caregivers to listen to accusations of theft or adultery targeted at them and then, calmly, try to help. Again, the psychiatrist can help the caregiver and the victim. If the paranoid ideas are very disruptive to the family, major tranquilizers are most beneficial to calm the agitation and reduce the intensity.

32

HALLUCINATIONS

Seeing, hearing, tasting, or smelling things that are not present are called *hallucinations*. Many individuals with Alzheimer's disease, perhaps one in two, experience hallucinations at some point during the illness. The phenomenon usually occurs from the middle stage onward. Hallucinations are rarely seen in the early stage. Individuals are not aware that they are having hallucinations, and many proceed to describe in great detail what they see. They tell you about people sitting at the dinner table or coming into the bedroom. These descriptions are usually quite realistic and detailed. They actually see a fully dressed and lively individual, often a family member or a friend.

It is important to understand that hallucinations are often pleasant; many Alzheimer's victims mention with delight "the people who visit every afternoon." Often they see a parent—a regression to early childhood. Hallucinations usually reflect *need states*. For instance, a lonely Alzheimer's victim may "need" to imagine the company of playing children, as during a more pleasant time of life. A woman with eight children, now all grown, often sees young children in her living room: this is both a sign of a need state and a memory of the past triggered by the lonely present.

These hallucinations are not constant. They may come and go during the day. Caregivers usually report them in the middle to late stages of the disease.

Hallucinations should be discussed with the physician because they can be a result of problems other than Alzheimer's disease. For instance, individuals may report smells, particularly of burnt garbage or other bad odors; this can be a sign of epileptic seizures (in the part of the brain known as the temporal lobe), which can be easily treated. The majority of hallucinations do not require treatment or drugs of any sort, however, and the individual can be left to enjoy the presence or the sounds of fictitious friends.

If hallucinations become disruptive and disturb necessary activities of daily living, such as eating or sleeping, major tranquilizers may be prescribed to help calm the individual and lessen the effect of the hallucinations.

The caregiver's role should be passive. It is most desirable to agree to the individual's statement and attempt to distract the individual by moving to another setting.

33

COMMUNICATION PROBLEMS

Anyone who comes in contact with an individual who suffers from Alzheimer's disease becomes acutely aware of communication problems. The individual has problems communicating, because he doesn't always understand what you are saying and doesn't remember what you just said. In addition, he often forgets a specific word to describe something and becomes increasingly frustrated as he attempts to make himself understood.

On the other hand, you may have real trouble communicating with the individual because you are becoming aware of her memory loss and her general limitations and you are in a quandary about what to discuss. Furthermore, your own anxiety, frustration, and anger build up and make communication more difficult.

Should you limit yourself to very plain statements that are not likely to trigger agitation? Or should you continue to challenge your loved one with stimulating intellectual conversation?

In the early stages of Alzheimer's disease, when memory loss is just being noticed, conversation should flow as always with no change in content or context. If a slight memory lapse occurs, the caregiver or family member can fill in the missing information, downplaying its importance. For example, Grandma may be talking with the children about the school curriculum, having forgotten that the oldest child is already in college. An appropriate statement might be, "Time moves so fast. Can you believe that John is now already in college?"

In the middle stages, the Alzheimer's victim becomes more confused and very repetitious. He will ask over and over again, "Where are my glasses?" Communication at this stage should be more passive. A quiet monologue about the holidays coming soon or the children's visit in the near future is much preferable to a two-way conversation with complex questions and answers. Keep the communication process simple and focused. Do not provide too much information because this only increases the confusion. Repetitive questions require infinite patience. Try to distract the patient by changing the setting or the situation. For instance, to the question, Where are my glasses?, you may want to show the individual his glasses, place them on his nose, and then suggest a nice walk or a cup of tea!

Remember that your body language is communication, too. If you act agitated, anxious, or frustrated, you raise the individual's anxiety level and escalate the situation into a confrontation. Act calm, even if you are upset. Speak in a low-pitched and slow voice. Avoid noisy settings that can distract and confuse the individual. The Alzheimer's victim is using all the brain power she has left to understand and communicate with you.

All outside stimulations and interference complicate your communication. Large group settings are not good for the individual with Alzheimer's. Concentrate on one-on-one interactions. Your telephone calls to the individual should be brief, with a single message at a time. On the other hand, expect your own phone to ring often. You may want to purchase an answering machine so that you can screen incoming phone calls. Make sure that your own recorded message states who you are and that you will soon return the call so that the individual is reassured by hearing the familiar sound of your voice. You may want to say, for instance, "This is Jeff. I can't answer your call right now, but I'll call you back as soon as I can. Please leave your message after the beep." Avoid background music, which is distracting and confusing.

Be aware that the individual can still understand much of what is being said. Do not discuss in front of him things you do not wish to make him aware of, and never talk about him with other people without including him in the conversation.

As the disease progresses, the individual may be less and less able to communicate her thoughts and needs. She may mumble incoherently or repeat syllables, as in "mamamama." You need to learn how to read her body language. Is she holding her head, indicating perhaps a headache? Is she pushing on her stomach because she has abdominal cramps from constipation?

It is more important than ever to communicate using very simple, one-level sentences. Do not use open-ended questions, which require a complex answering process. If you are planning to go to the supermarket, tell the individual, "We are going shopping," rather than "I have to pick up milk and vegetables on my way to the hairdresser. Would you like to come along?" Accept that your loved one's vocabulary is decreasing as he is forgetting words. Let him point to objects rather than describe them.

Above all, remember that one doesn't need words to communicate caring and love. A hug, a smile, and a pat on the shoulder convey the warmth of your affection better than any speech.

34

WHEN TO USE
TRANQUILIZERS

The individual with Alzheimer's disease is likely to exhibit periods of anxiety and agitation. (See Key 30.) Often these moments represent deep frustration about the inability to remember and genuine fright at the lack of memory clues for the next action they are supposed to take. In general, Alzheimer's victims are rarely physically abusive, particularly against children. They tend to ignore younger children and focus more on themselves unless unduly distracted and forced into an unwanted activity. Additionally, in the early stage, the individual generally shows signs of depression, because his or her judgment of the situation is not yet impaired. This depression, which lasts until the individual's judgment fails, responds to antidepressants.

For the treatment of agitation and anxiety, tranquilizers are helpful medications. However, they do not treat or cure the source of these symptoms, which is the Alzheimer's process itself. Because tranquilizers are geared only at *easing* symptoms, they should be used only when symptoms are discomforting to the victim or family. In other words, not every symptom of agitation requires a tranquilizer.

Historically, tranquilizers have been divided into minor and major categories.

Minor Tranquilizers

Minor tranquilizers, such as Ativan®, Valium®, and Xanax®, and sedatives, such as Dalmane® and Restoril®, have been used to control anxiety, slight agitation, and insomnia. These are by and large safe and commonly prescribed. They can produce side effects, however, such as increased confusion, further memory impairment, and loss of balance, and they are potentially addictive.

Major Tranquilizers

The major tranquilizers (Haldol®, Mellaril®, and Navane®) are used to reduce the intensity of psychotic symptoms, such as hallucinations, delusions, and paranoid ideas. Unfortunately, all these drugs have serious side effects, the most feared being *tardive dyskinesia* (TD), a syndrome that manifests itself by involuntary tic movements, particularly of the mouth area. Patients may smack the lips, stick out the tongue uncontrollably, or appear to be chewing food constantly. This side effect is more likely after long-term use of these drugs.

In addition, major tranquilizers do not make the psychotic symptoms disappear but rather decrease their intensity.

Their use should be reserved for hallucinations that are frightening to the Alzheimer's victim and highly disturbing to the family. An example of this behavior is Mrs. A.G., who believed she saw a monster every time she looked in the mirror. She would proceed to hit the mirror and injure herself on the broken glass. Her family was forced to cover every mirror in the house, but reflections in windows produced the same reaction. Major tranquilizers were needed to treat this individual. Individuals who experience pleasant or nonbothersome delusions, such as imagining nice people sitting in the living room for coffee and cake, should not be medicated. (See Key 32.)

35

DEPRESSION

Depression occurs often in individuals with Alzheimer's disease. Some studies report that over half of Alzheimer's victims suffer from major depression, expressed as hopelessness, sadness, loss of sleep, loss of appetite, and poor concentration. The individual may develop feelings of guilt and even think of committing suicide.

Depression occurs in Alzheimer's disease for two reasons:
1. A cellular cause: the degeneration of the brain cell itself.
2. An intellectual cause: the realization by patients that they have a chronic dementing illness.

First, let's address the changes in the brain. *Neurotransmitters*, chemical substances responsible for the normal function of the brain, are reduced in aging. Many of these neurotransmitters, such as norepinephrine and serotonin, are also implicated in the development of depression. Therefore, normal aging in itself raises the potential of developing depression and reduces our ability to cope as well as we did when we were younger. With degenerative brain disease, such as Alzheimer's disease, there is further damage to the neurotransmitter cells, which increases even more the risk of developing depression.

Second, in the early stages of the disease, the individual may realize that he or she is developing memory trouble. (See Key 6.) This is a worrisome discovery. Anxiety and depression may ensue. In fact, one of the initial signs of Alzheimer's disease is often the onset of a depressed mood. The patient may appear sad, unusually quiet, or unwilling to participate in family activities.

In addition to these two simultaneous processes, the aging individual may be at risk for depression because of other factors, such as facing retirement or loss of siblings and social support. Recently, a well-known scientist came to us for evaluation of memory loss and depression. All his life he was revered by his colleagues and family for his outstanding accomplishments. He now faced retirement because of his age and was very fearful of his future, without his work, his colleagues, his secretarial help, and his library. Was this man truly suffering from Alzheimer's disease, or was his memory loss a result of his untreated depression? Probably both, and both should be addressed.

The memory is involved with all intellectual processes. If one's self-esteem is based on memory, a realization of this precious loss may increase the feelings of loss of self-worth: I am no good anymore. I can't even remember what I did yesterday. Individuals who have stressed the need to perform at a high level all their lives and can no longer function at that level because of memory loss have a tendency to develop serious depression.

How should one respond to depression? Seek advice fast. (See Key 9.) Depression can worsen the preexisting memory loss because the individual won't even bother to try to remember. The memory loss can be temporarily improved by appropriate treatment of the depression. The treatment should consist of a thorough evaluation by a psychiatrist, a geriatrician, or a well-trained physician. (See Key 10.) Other causes for depression, such as underlying medical illnesses, should be looked for and treated.

At this stage, antidepressant medications, such as desipramine (Norpramin®), nortriptyline (Aventyl®, Pamelor®), or bupropion hydrochloride (Wellbutrin®), should be started in small doses. The choice of medication is based on the specific pharmacological action of each drug. (See Key 14.) Some of them are calming and sedating, better suited for the agitated, depressed patient who has trouble falling asleep. Desyrel® (trazodone) is one example in this category. Other antidepressants, such as Wellbutrin® and Prozac®, affect different chemicals in the brain and alleviate the depression without producing sedation.

Antidepressants can cause dizziness upon standing, constipation, dryness of mouth, and blurred vision. They can also increase the risk of having a seizure if one has a history of seizure disorder and may cause more confusion and irritability. For the treatment of depression, *small doses* of antianxiety agents, such as lorazepam (Ativan®) and alprazolam (Xanax®), can be helpful. The rule of thumb when treating elderly people is to start with low doses and increase the dose slowly. In many cases, expect to see results in weeks, not days. Also be aware that 30 percent of patients with major depression do not respond to medication. These patients continue to refuse food and are unable to sleep, endangering their own lives. At that point an aggressive medical treatment is needed, which must act fast. The therapy of choice is electroconvulsive therapy (ECT). ECT is one of the safest and most effective treatments available. It can be literally a lifesaver, especially for those individuals who neither respond to antidepressant medication nor can tolerate some of the side effects of the drugs.

Furthermore, one of the best ways to ease anxiety and ward off depression is through structure: a day-care program providing activities and companionship might greatly improve the individual's outlook. Family support is possibly the most important aspect of the therapeutic approach. (See Key 22.) The caregiver bears the awesome burden of helping the loved one deal with this condition. If the individual perceives ambivalence or open hostility on the part of the family, he or she may become even more depressed!

The most important point is to *expect* depression, to look for it, and to be willing to seek treatment for it.

36

URINARY AND FECAL INCONTINENCE

Incontinence is an involuntary loss of urine or stools. Incontinence usually happens in an inappropriate setting, that is, outside a bathroom. Many elderly people develop incontinence as they age. Women who have had multiple pregnancies are at particular risk for developing some degree of urinary incontinence. Often they wear sanitary napkins or a pad to avoid soiling their clothes. Some women have learned to go to the bathroom very frequently, perhaps every two to three hours, to avoid accumulating large amounts of urine inside the bladder. Elderly males with prostate enlargement also develop urinary frequency because they cannot completely evacuate the bladder. Urine may dribble.

If these people develop Alzheimer's disease, they of course continue to have urinary incontinence. However, Alzheimer's disease in itself does not cause urinary or fecal incontinence until the very last stages of the disease, when the victim, now bedridden, loses all control over bodily functions.

Most Alzheimer's sufferers in the early to moderate stages have no problem with urinary incontinence provided they remember where the toilet is. In fact, most "accidents" are a result of inaccessibility to bathrooms or clumsy clothing.

If a new pattern of urinary incontinence develops, a medical evaluation can determine whether there is a bladder infection, which can be treated, or another easily remedied cause. Comprehensive *urodynamic studies*, an exam of the urinary tract, from the kidney to the urethra, including the bladder, should not be undertaken if no specific treatment, such as surgery, will be carried out because of the individual's mental condition.

As a rule, it is best to anticipate the individual's need using the toilet by adhering to a convenient schedule, after meals and before bedtime. The bathroom door should be left open as a visual clue to the individual. Clothes should be fitted with convenient, easy-to-open fasteners such as Velcro®. Use specific communication techniques when you want to take a moderately demented individual to the toilet. Take the individual by the arm, place your arm under his, and inform him, "We are going to the bathroom." Do not ask if he wants to go, because then you open the door to "No!" Walk with the individual into the stall and help pull his pants down. Jogging pants with elastic waistbands are very convenient. Encourage the individual to sit while you run water at the sink. Stay to offer reassurance, and talk in a calm manner about what you will do as soon as he has finished voiding or defecating. Use wet wipes if you can. They are much more convenient for you and for the Alzheimer's victim. Offer toilet tissue.

As urinary and/or stool incontinence appears, it is helpful to deal with this in a concrete and practical manner. Incontinence is very stressful for the caregiver and is one of the leading causes for institutionalization. In addition, urine or stool leakage can create skin irritation and discomfort to the individual and lead to possible further agitation.

Drug treatment for incontinence is not very helpful in these individuals. We recommend incontinence undergarments and pads and, in special circumstances, catheters.

Undergarments and Pads

In the past decade, industry has responded to the needs of the millions of incontinent persons, who have created a market for "adult diapers." These undergarments can be found in regular supermarkets, usually with the feminine hygiene products and the sanitary napkin displays. All these products contain absorbent material designed to keep the skin dry. Because they are somewhat cumbersome, they should not be used for infrequent episodes of incontinence but rather for the more advanced stages when the individual is no longer able to attempt to go to the bathroom on his or her own.

Purchase adult diapers in the local supermarket or surgical supply store. They come in small, medium, and large sizes. Most of them have adhesive tape that can be refastened, a plus when the diaper you check is dry. Make sure the tape is never fastened to the individual's skin. Change the diaper whenever needed. At each change, make sure that the skin is left clean and dry to avoid the development of sores.

If the individual oozes feces, he or she may be fecally impacted, which means so constipated that he or she cannot push out a stool. This can be dangerous. Stools may have to be removed manually (manual disimpaction) or even surgically. Keep track of the regularity of bowel movements. There is no need for daily evacuation. However, if five to seven days has elapsed since the last bowel movement, contact the physician. An enema and/or laxatives might be needed. Remember that good *hydration* —at least eight glasses of water a day—is essential to normal bowel movements.

Catheters

Plastic tubes can be placed inside the bladder by the physician or a visiting nurse and linked to a plastic container that can be emptied periodically. The tubes are left in for several weeks and changed as needed. Unfortunately, these tubes, or *catheters*, can cause serious urinary tract infections because bacteria can penetrate the bladder more easily.

The physician may recommend the use of a Texas condom catheter for men; these are external devices, rolled directly onto the penis and linked to a container by a tube. There is a risk of discomfort, damage to the penis itself, and possible infection. There is no similar device for women.

Because of the risk of infection, catheters should not be used routinely but left to the judgment of the physician.

37

I CAN'T STAND IT ANYMORE!

You will experience times of complete frustration and despair. This is normal and is expected. Anticipate these times by preparing for such an eventuality. As a rule, do not expect family or friends to help out. Prepare your own "emergency plan." Your relatives will be much more supportive if they do not feel put upon. Furthermore, their advice, particularly in times of crisis, may not always be sound. Here are some steps you should consider.

- Talk to the physician about emergency placement in your town. Most cities have an emergency center for short-term hospitalization of individuals with Alzheimer's while problems at home are resolved. This may be a lifesaver if you must undergo unexpected surgery or take a sudden trip, or if you feel you are on the verge of a nervous breakdown. In the worse-case scenario, you can always call the emergency police number (911, where it is available) to transport the Alzheimer's victim to the nearest hospital for placement. Obviously, this is a last resort.

- Explore through community resources and especially the local Alzheimer's Association chapter the local *respite* programs. These programs accept the Alzheimer's victim during the day, usually for a modest fee per hour. This respite time allows you freedom to catch up on daily errands or visit with friends—or rest! The local Alzheimer's Association chapter may be able to help you find out about short-term overnight respite programs which are not affiliated with hospitals.

- Consider hiring a home health care attendant who will come on a regular basis. Begin looking before you are desperate! This gives you a chance to select the right person without pressure and to observe the interaction. Expect, at first, reticence and suspicion on the part of the Alzheimer's victim. The attendant is someone new, unknown, and unfamiliar. With time, this attitude will change and you will feel comfortable leaving the caretaker for prolonged periods of time.

- Plan regular "vacations" for yourself. This is the time to ask the caretaker and family members to take over for a few days while you treat yourself to a trip.
- Attend local support groups. The Alzheimer's Association offers groups for spouses and for children of Alzheimer's victims. Sharing your feelings with others in similar situations helps a great deal! You might find common solutions.
- Accept seeing a psychiatrist for a few sessions of psychotherapy. Feelings of anger, frustration, despair, and depression should be explored and discussed with professionals who are trained in helping you deal with them. They should not be forced on family members, who may or may not be willing or able to provide support. Your physician can give you a referral to a qualified psychiatrist.

38

GUILT

Guilt affects every family member of the Alzheimer's victim, and the individual with the disease.

Patient's Guilt

In the early to moderate stages of the disease, some Alzheimer's victims feel guilty: "I am going to become a burden on my family." In the later stages, as insight and judgment diminish, guilt disappears. To ease the feelings of guilt, these individuals should discuss these concerns with the doctor, who can help by reviewing constructive steps to be taken at this point. For example, this is a good time to finalize financial and legal matters, to discuss eventual nursing home placement, and to arrange for home help. It is also a time to enjoy life to the fullest and renew family ties.

Spouse's Guilt

The spouse is the most likely person to suffer from the overwhelming burden of guilt. It is the spouse who shares the life and the home of the victim and is exposed on an hourly basis to the progressive deterioration in memory and judgment. Reactions include frustration, anger, and sometimes verbal and physical abuse. Attempts to leave the patient for a few hours to take care of shopping errands are met with increased hostility and agitation upon return. These reactions are intensified by the constant, unrelenting dependency manifested by the Alzheimer's victim. Most individuals with advanced Alzheimer's disease literally follow their spouse around the house. The spouse feels trapped in assuming the complete responsibility for this now totally helpless human being.

The guilt felt by the spouse may also be related to the nature of the relationship. If the relationship was based on love and caring, the reaction of guilt is not as strong. If, on the other hand, the relationship was a poor one or at best ambivalent, guilt may rear its ugly head: Now I have to take care of this woman whom I thought about leaving before. The caregiver's reaction at best is conflicted and, at worst, verbally or physically abusive.

Consideration of nursing home placement becomes one more guilt-producing matter. Support for the spouse can be obtained through the Alzheimer's Association (800-272-3900, Monday through Friday).

Guilt of Other Family Members

Sometimes, one child assumes responsibility for the parent, stimulating guilt and anger on the part of other siblings. The very diagnosis of Alzheimer's disease may be disputed by other siblings, who believe—and say so!—that the deterioration is a result of poor care rather than an intrinsic pathological process. Often, the responsible sibling becomes the object of blame. The child providing care to the Alzheimer's victim becomes resentful as he or she is saddled with this new responsibility in addition to already existing pressures in his or her own family and career. Awareness of family dynamics is very helpful. For example, the child caregiver may be subconsciously trying to win the parent's greater love by showing more consideration and interest. Noninvolved siblings may actually fear the possible hereditary effects of the disease and would rather ignore its existence. In addition, as described earlier, the spouse's reaction to the illness and the relationship of the children to their parent with Alzheimer's depend on their relationships before the illness. Reactions range from I don't care and Leave me out of it to complete devotion and dedication—to the neglect of other responsibilities. Professional counseling is recommended for such family difficulties. Your physician is probably the best source of referral.

39

COMMUNITY RESOURCES

Thanks to the growing public awareness of Alzheimer's disease, several organizations have sprouted up throughout the country to assist and educate relatives of Alzheimer's victims. The largest program is the Alzheimer's Association, which is based in Chicago. It was started in 1980 and has over 200 chapters. The telephone number is 800-621-0379 (Monday through Friday). They offer a comprehensive listing of community resources in your area.

Besides the nursing agencies who provide paid help, several volunteer agencies may be of assistance. Check with the local churches or temples. Many have home visitor programs that give you respite. Visit the senior citizens center; they have a wealth of information for you.

You can also call the local department of aging for programs they offer. You can find the telephone number in the directory or at the local library. Look for bulletin board announcements in the library, bank, or supermarket.

Finally, call the nearest medical center and ask for the telephone number of the geriatric division or department. The division is usually linked to the department of internal medicine, the department of family practice, or the department of psychiatry. At the geriatric department, you will find a social worker who can give you direct information about available services and their cost.

Be aware, once again, that Medicare, for which you qualify when you reach the age of 65, does not pay for long-term care. In other words, the costs of a home attendant, of a respite program, and of a nursing home are not covered by Medicare. As federal and state regulations change often, you should attempt to contact your local representative of governmental and other agencies. Medicare information can be obtained by dialing 1-800-772-1213. Local agencies on Aging can be contacted by the National Association of Area Agencies on Aging (NAAAA) 202-296-8130. You are expected to pay for these services privately, unless you obtain private long-term insurance plans. However, you may qualify for Medicaid if your monthly income is low. The criteria for qualification, based on your financial assets, vary from state to state. As you spend your money reserves, you might reach eligibility for Medicaid support. (See Appendix for Additional Resources.)

40

DAY CARE AND RESPITE CARE

Day-care programs for elderly people have developed in the past decade. Originally started to help veterans of World War II receive physical therapy to reintegrate into the work force, they are now available to many different groups, including handicapped and elderly persons. These programs are usually available during the day, Monday through Friday, and offer socialization, nutritious meals, and activities. Some of them add medical and rehabilitation services. These medical or psychosocial models provide care for people with various diseases or frailties. Many of these individuals have had strokes or have heart problems. The goal of these programs is to provide a social setting for recreational activities and entertainment to fight loneliness. Within the program, some medical or nursing supervision can be provided. These programs can accommodate Alzheimer's victims in the early stage of the disease.

Unfortunately, staffing does not allow one-on-one care. Unless the individual is very fit and still able to participate in group activities, he or she will not do well in this kind of program. Wandering and behavioral problems exclude an individual from participation. Discuss your specific needs with the director of the program, and see how they can be accommodated.

Most people with Alzheimer's disease do better in a specific *dementia day-care program*. Therefore, sooner or later, you may wish to move on to an Alzheimer's respite center or day program for individuals with Alzheimer's. In contrast to day care, these programs are exclusively geared to the needs of demented elderly people. Dementia day care involves an area that is usually proofed against wandering. A "rest room" is provided to allow agitated individuals to calm down in a quiet setting. The pace is less hectic, and the staff anticipates behavioral challenges. Also, the other participants do not react to the individual's confusion and repetitious speech. Most of these Alzheimer's day-care programs offer many services to caregivers in addition to the victims themselves. They often organize support groups and informative lectures. They also have access to community resources and can network for you.

Ask about transportation. It will be very helpful for you to know that the individual can be picked up and returned to your home while you catch up on rest or handle household chores. Also, inquire about the ratio of staff to clients. Although individualized attention is good, it is not always achievable because of the cost. One staff member to three or four clients is a very acceptable ratio.

You will be tempted to stay with the individual. Learn to trust the staff, and leave the center. They know how to handle the Alzheimer's victim, and you need the break. This is time for you to enjoy and relax.

Don't think that you are the only one who can handle your demented relative. The fact that he or she follows you everywhere, every minute, is an indication that memory and judgment are lost, not that *you* are indispensable to his or her survival. Often a demented individual follows anyone who is pleasant and reassuring. The staff who provide care in Alzheimer's day programs are compassionate and caring; they have chosen to work in these settings rather than in other health care fields or businesses. Also, because they are not as closely related to the victim as you are, they are less likely to become frustrated or angered by the individual's behavior. If you relinquish a portion of the responsibility for caregiving, even for a few hours, you will actually feel better able to cope when your loved one returns to your care.

41

HOW TO FIND A GOOD HOME ATTENDANT

Before you look for the perfect caretaker, sit back and think of what you need this person to do. The priorities should be (1) to relate well to the individual with Alzheimer's, (2) exert a calming influence and prevent potential injury, (3) provide personal hygiene care, including bathing, helping to the toilet, grooming, and dressing, and (4) prepare simple but nutritious meals.

Do not expect the caretaker to take charge of your household, your children, or your pets.

To find the right person, you can either contact an agency or seek a caretaker through friends, family, church, or other sources. A very helpful resource book is *Caring for an Alzheimer's Disease Patient at Home*, by Shulman and Steinberg (Fidia Pharmaceutical Corp.), 1988, distributed by the New York City chapter of the Alzheimer's Association (551 Fifth Avenue, NY, NY 10176, Phone 212-983-0700).

Home Care Agencies

These agencies charge a fee to arrange a selection of trained home attendants. Possible problems can be referred to the agency supervisor, and emergency replacement is handled. When you contact the agency, you need the answers to several questions:

1. Costs of services, including travel time for the attendant.
2. Screening and training protocols for attendants.
3. Crisis situations: Who covers accidents in the home? Are employees bonded for theft? What happens if the attendant doesn't show up?

Make sure that you know the name of the supervisor and how to contact that person at any time. Ask for references.

Self-Referral

Local sources of home attendants include the local newspaper, supermarket bulletin board, church or temple volunteer group, friends, and neighbors. When you interview potential caretakers, obtain at least one recent reference and check that reference. Have the person meet the Alzheimer's victim. Note any hesitancy, expression of fear, or uneasiness on the part of the caretaker. Observe the pace of the speech and of the actions.

Individuals with Alzheimer's do better with calm people. Beware of long fingernails! Washing and helping an agitated person to the toilet require short fingernails to avoid scratches. Plan to spend at least the first two sessions with the home attendant, familiarizing him or her with your loved one's preferences and rehearsing emergency procedures (fire, police, doctor, and ambulance). Don't be surprised if the Alzheimer's sufferer rejects the "intruder" at first. Work to help the caretaker acclimate to the household, so that the individual with Alzheimer's eventually feels that he or she is part of the family.

A realistic beginning schedule should include at least three or four hours, two to three times a week. This can be progressively increased to accommodate your needs.

If the Alzheimer's sufferer asks you why this person is here, respond, "Because she helps me in the house." Do not be surprised if paranoid feelings surge. After assuring yourself that the accusations are unfounded, express your support to the home attendant and discuss the paranoia with the doctor.

42

WHEN TO CONSIDER NURSING HOME PLACEMENT

The decision on nursing home placement is a dynamic process that rests on your needs and the Alzheimer's sufferer's demands.

Your Needs

Face reality! How much can you take? Are you prepared to accept a home attendant in your life, to trust such a person, while you take short breaks and true vacations, to remain healthy medically and physically? Are you running out of energy, of stamina? Have you reached the point where you fear you may become physically abusive to your loved one when he or she repeats themselves and follows you everywhere? Have you lost all contact with your friends because your life revolves exclusively around the Alzheimer's victim? If so, *you* are ready for nursing home placement. This is not a failure on your part but rather a mature decision process that makes you select the best option for you.

The Individual's Demands

As long as an individual is aware of the surroundings, recognizes his or her room, and goes to the kitchen or to the bathroom purposefully, he or she should probably be kept at home.

Unfortunately, many individuals eventually forget where they are. In fact, they may beg to "go home" while sitting in their own living rooms! They might remember the home of childhood as "home" rather than the house they have lived in during their married lives. These individuals are ready to be transferred to a nursing home if you are ready.

This is a very critical personal decision which depends on a multiplicity of factors and conditions. There are no right and wrong answers. Emotional issues as well as physical and financial considerations must be weighted. In addition, the Alzheimer's victim may be developing physical problems such as incontinence, unsafe gait with recurrent falls, inability to swallow, and perhaps bedsores. You may not be able to handle these problems and the Alzheimer's sufferer would do better in a skilled nursing facility.

43

HOW TO SELECT A GOOD NURSING HOME

The nursing home industry has received a lot of bad press because of some cases of abuse and neglect. By and large, the industry is now closely monitored by state and federal inspectors. Cleanliness of the building facilities, food preparation, medication usage and resident's satisfaction are key items reviewed on a regular basis. Quality of life issues are viewed by state and federal agencies on an equal par with medical care issues. Failure to pass established standards of care leads to financial and administrative penalties.

When you are ready to select a nursing home, choose one near your home so that you can visit as often as you want. If you do not know of any, call the local hospital and ask for the discharge planning program and the home care program. Both programs have either a nurse or a social worker on the staff who can suggest nursing homes in the area. The local department on aging or department of health can also furnish a list of nursing homes in the community. Another option is to visit the library and ask for a reference book—a directory of nursing homes.

Call the nursing home, and make an appointment with the admission staff person to visit the place. Ask to see the most recent annual survey by state agencies. You should know which deficiencies were found on the survey, such as dietary problems or nursing care issues, and what was done to correct these deficiencies. Does the nursing home have a residents' council that meets periodically? Are minutes available of these meetings? Ask about residents' rights and responsibilities. Is the residents' bill of rights prominently displayed in public locations? Can you easily locate the telephone number for the ombudsman program, should a problem arise? What are the visiting hours? Are children and pets welcome?

Get a general feel for the building. Is it clean? Does it smell of urine or feces? Do the employees appear cheerful and talkative?

If at all possible, speak to some of the nurses and orderlies: find out how long they have been working in the nursing home and how long on a specific floor. Does the nursing staff interact with the residents? Do the residents talk to each other, or do they sit alone? What is the noise level on the units? What use is made of television sets? How are the residents dressed and groomed? Are they encouraged to wear their own clothes? How often are laundry services provided? Are you expected to do some of the laundry? Ask to see a menu: is it varied and appealing?

Look at the activities schedule: how often are programs scheduled? Try to attend a program of activities in session. Are the residents enjoying themselves? Is the therapist stimulating and personable? What activities are specifically available for Alzheimer's victims? Inquire about the services of a chaplain. Are religious services available at the nursing home? Is there a quiet space for families to visit privately with their loved ones?

Do not overlook fire and safety. Can you easily locate the exit signs?

Inquire about policies regarding medical emergencies. To which hospital will your loved one be transferred if a problem arises? Ask specifically about policies on physical and chemical restraints (tranquilizers). Are these routinely ordered for individuals with Alzheimer's? How will the staff notify you and discuss with you the need for restraints should it arise?

You have the right to participate in your loved one's care-planning process. Find out how you will be able to give your input and how you will get feedback. Inquire about Do Not Resuscitate (DNR) (see Key 48) policies and tube feeding arrangements.

Some nursing homes have special units geared to Alzheimer's victims; they may have wanderproof doors, home-like furniture, and specially trained staff members. Not all individuals are admitted to such a unit; find out the selection criteria.

Last but not least, check on the procedure for admission. How long is the waiting list (it is not unusual to wait four to six months for a bed), and what are the charges (an initial deposit of several thousand dollars is often requested to cover the cost of the nursing home until insurance or Medicaid payments arrive)? What will these charges cover? Will your insurance cover any of these expenses? What happens if the individual is discharged from the nursing home: are unspent monies returned to you? Try to get as much information as possible in writing.

To help you decide between nursing homes, make a list of *your* priorities. No home will be absolutely perfect! If your most pressing needs can be met (for instance, location, clean-liness, and affordability), you should feel that you have done your homework conscientiously and you should be satisfied with your choice.

44

WHEN TO VISIT THE NURSING HOME

Once your loved one has been admitted to the nursing home, you may be anxious to visit often and for prolonged periods of time. There is usually no objection to your doing so, but the goals of institutionalization are to provide you with some free time, as well as to ensure good quality of care for the resident.

Therefore, after the initial week of adjustment, we suggest that you consider spacing your visits, perhaps to every other day or every third day.

If the nursing home is conveniently located and you have no access problem, you may want to come to visit every day for short periods of time. Ask the nursing staff when they prefer you to visit. If baths are given in the morning, the afternoon may be a better time. Some nurses welcome your help during feeding times, at lunch or at dinner, when less staff is available.

Other nursing homes would rather have you visit on weekends, when the program of therapeutic activities may be lighter and the residents less busy with scheduled entertainment.

Be aware that the change in nursing shifts is a particularly hectic time. There are usually three shifts, the daytime (8 A.M. to 4 P.M.), the evening (4 P.M. to midnight), and the night (midnight to 8 A.M.) During the transition, nurses for both shifts meet and report on the resident's condition and progress. This is not a good time for you to visit.

What to Do if You Get Sick

Occasionally, there are outbreaks of influenza and other viral illnesses in the community. These occur frequently during the months of February or March. During these periods, the administration may request that you temporarily suspend your visits to avoid bringing in germs. As a rule, do not visit if you are coming down with a cold. Check with the head nurse on the unit about how to get information on your loved one; there is usually someone on the floor who can give you information by telephone.

45

HOW TO VISIT THE NURSING HOME

Contact with the Nursing Home Staff

Nursing homes are staffed and run by people. Some of them are very good; some of them show less compassion and less concern. Mistakes can occur, just as they might occur in your home, because no one can be expected to provide nonstop 24 hour individual attention.

You may be tempted to focus on details that displease you or on a staff member who did not display the courtesy you expect. This reaction on your part is natural and is explained by your eagerness to reassure yourself that you made the right decision in choosing this nursing home. A more constructive approach is to focus on those findings that are positive—the warmth and understanding of one nurse or a well-prepared meal or stimulating activity. Praise the staff who continue to attempt to provide excellent nursing care. Support them, and they will support you. If you experience difficulty, discuss it calmly with the nurse at a convenient time for both of you. Do not become aggravated if you have a communication problem; a nursing supervisor can help you. Find out who he or she is through the nursing office. Remember that most nursing homes organize nursing care in three shifts around the clock: 8 A.M. to 4 P.M., 4 P.M. to midnight, and midnight to 8 A.M. If a problem seems to be occurring mostly in the evening, you want the name of the evening nursing supervisor.

Meet the social worker on the unit. Social workers are trained to help you adjust to emotional crises, and their expertise may be helpful. If you feel that you have a serious complaint that is not being handled appropriately by the nursing home, contact the nursing home ombudsman program. Your local office on aging has the telephone number. The ombudsman program can investigate the problem for you.

Most nursing homes do not allow tipping. Often a smile, a compliment, or perhaps even a complimentary letter addressed to a supervisor is more rewarding than tipping.

Contact with Residents

Be cheerful, calm, and positive. Share news about the family; bring along pictures and recent letters. Talk about familiar events, workplace, church, or temple. Tell them about your life and your interests. Avoid quizzing them, which is frustrating. By and large, do not contradict them.

If allowed, bring along a child and a pet. Even if the Alzheimer's victim is not sure who the child is, he or she is likely to smile and react to the child. Remember, however, that neither the child nor the patient has a great deal of tolerance or patience! Shorten your visit to accommodate both their needs.

Many nursing homes encourage your bringing familiar objects from the resident's home. In our experience, most individuals with Alzheimer's disease have forgotten "memories" by the time they enter a nursing home. A treasured heirloom is probably safer in your own living room than on the resident's nightstand. However, a light blanket or a familiar quilt may provide a feeling of security and warmth.

It is also a good idea to take food or a sweet treat. Hard candies may be dangerous because the individual can choke on them. Check with the nurse about whether you have permission to feed the patient. Try to select items that are not too messy, such as cakes or cookies. Ice cream in the summer is usually very welcome.

Ask whether you can take the individual on outings for the day. If you do so, consider hiring an aide who will help you with the transfer into the car and perhaps in taking the resident to the toilet. Outings include trips to the park, to the hair salon, to a family restaurant, or to a close friend's house. Make sure you have medications with you if they have been prescribed.

A question often asked by well-meaning and caring family members is how to plan a visit at holiday time or for family occasions. Although it is a nice idea to continue involving the Alzheimer's victim in family life, there might be too much excitement and stimulation during that event for the good of the individual. This may ruin the party for you and for others. If you are determined that the individual attend the party, consider hiring a paid companion and selecting a quiet room where the individual and the companion can retire should the event be too anxiety provoking. As a rule, a visit to the nursing home with a few selected friends and family members after the event is usually the best approach for the resident and for you.

46

HOW TO FIND AN ATTORNEY

Alzheimer's disease is a chronic and costly illness. We recommend that you find a good attorney to resolve legal and financial situations as soon as possible. In the early stages of Alzheimer's disease, even though memory loss is obvious, the individual's *judgment* is not impaired. Hence, decisions can be made by the victim about who should control the finances, who should be responsible for his or her ultimate care, and where this care should take place. Financial trusts can often be created to save considerable expense. Because tax laws change frequently, an experienced lawyer, familiar with elder care issues, needs to be consulted.

There are several sources of referral. The best is word of mouth. Talk to your friends and neighbors. Meet with other spouses of Alzheimer's victims in local support groups of the Alzheimer's Association. Find out who they use for legal counseling. Many lawyers interested in geriatric problems volunteer their services and speak at community meetings. Plan to attend their conferences and get a first-hand idea of their style and knowledge.

You may have used an attorney in the past. He or she may not specialize in elder care issues but may be able to recommend someone with this special expertise.

You can certainly contact the local bar association. Check specifically for members of the disability or health care section and the trusts and estates section. Your local Alzheimer's Association chapter of the Department for the Aging Alzheimer's Resource Center can provide you with a list of attorneys.

Finally, you will find at the public library the *Martindale-Hubbell Directory*, which lists attorneys who are licensed to practice in your state. The listing provides the name of the attorney, year of graduation from law school, publications, and affiliations with firms. A small bibliography may give you the information you need on the specialization of the firm. Another useful book is the *National Academy of Elderlaw Attorneys*, which can be ordered from 655 North Alvernon, Suite 108, Tuscon, AZ 85711.

47

POWER OF ATTORNEY AND HEALTH CARE PROXY

You and I can decide how much medical care we want to receive, how far we want to go, and when we want to stop treatment because our minds are clear and we are deemed competent to make such decisions.

When a person is *no longer competent*, that is, no longer has a clear mind and good judgment in the eyes of the law, then this person's wishes concerning medical care can only be honored if there is clear and convincing evidence that this person's views on a course of medical action have been expressed. There are now several ways of creating such advance directives for health care.

To be prepared for the possibility that you may develop Alzheimer's disease or otherwise become incompetent, it is essential that you designate a responsible person whose task it will be to make decisions that you or your loved one can no longer make.

A *durable power of attorney* gives the person you designate the right to handle all your financial affairs, and this right holds even if you become incapacitated (hence, durable). By adding a paragraph, you can extend this right to the handling of other personal matters, including health care.

A durable power of attorney form can be purchased at stationery stores. The form with your signature must be *notarized* (certified by a notary public). You may want to leave a copy of this form with your bank officer or other fiscal agents.

Because of the complexity of the issues in dealing with Alzheimer's victims, we strongly recommend that you consider contacting an attorney to finalize paperwork and avoid possible problems in the future.

A new law in New York State allows you to officially appoint a designated person known as a *health care agent* by signing a document called the health care proxy. This form is available in all hospitals and nursing homes and from the state department of health. To fill out this form, you do not need a lawyer, only two adult witnesses. Keep copies of this document, and give copies to family members and to the doctor to avoid disruption of your intentions at a later stage. Once again, this decision to appoint a health care proxy can only be made by an alert and competent individual and should therefore be made in advance of any crisis. Your health care proxy agent can make any of the decisions you could have made regarding your medical treatment, except tube feeding and fluids. If you know now that you do not want such feeding, you must give the health care agent "clear and convincing evidence" of this, preferably in writing, and including the circumstances under which tube nutrition and hydration are to be withheld or withdrawn. By identifying the person you trust the most to make decisions on your behalf, you clarify, simplify, and assure the implementation of your plan of medical care. You may change or even cancel your health care proxy at any time that you remain able to make your own decisions. Your health care agent acts in your behalf only when you are not able to do so yourself.

48

ADVANCE DIRECTIVES AND THE DO NOT RESUSCITATE LAW

Living Wills

A *living will* is a legal document that permits you to make decisions regarding your health care over a broad range of issues. Its intent is to inform physicians of the medical treatment you would choose if you were to become terminally or hopelessly ill and could no longer communicate your intentions. The form must be completed when you are competent and able to make decisions. To avoid any possible challenge at a later date, we suggest that you have a medical examination at the time you execute a living will. (Similarly, a medical examination at the time of your health care proxy can confirm your competence to complete this advance directive.)

In the living will, you should leave instructions that are as specific as possible about the extent of medical care you want if you are in a terminal, a permanently unconscious, or a totally nonfunctional mental (vegetative) condition and can no longer speak for yourself. You can specify that you do not want cardiopulmonary resuscitation (CPR) when your heart stops beating or when you stop breathing. You can also specify whether you want chemotherapy, antibiotics, surgical interventions, or ventilation by respirator. A critical issue is whether you want to be fed and hydrated by artificial means (intravenous lines or tubes in your stomach).

A living will can be written on a plain piece of paper, but we suggest that you use a standard form, such as the one provided by Choice in Dying, Inc. (212-366-5540; see Appendix: Advance Directive). Make sure you have at least one witness's signature. This organization also has specific forms available for those states that have living will statutes. Your

119

state health department can also provide you with this form. The living will is most useful in the states that recognize it as a legal instrument. In other states, however, it serves to provide important information to be used as clear and convincing evidence of your choices.

Do Not Resuscitate (DNR)

The *do not resuscitate law*, issued in New York State in April 1989, allows you to make a decision regarding heroic measures at the time of your impending death. You can state that you do not want cardiopulmonary resuscitation.

The doctors perform CPR by pumping the chest to restore cardiac function and by introducing a tube into the lungs to connect you to a breathing machine and thereby bring oxygen to the lungs.

As you think through your decision for DNR, discuss with the physician your chances of surviving cardiopulmonary resuscitation. If you suffer from a progressive degenerative disease like Alzheimer's, it is extremely unlikely that your brain would resume any gratifying level of function because of intensive medical action after the heart has stopped.

If you are no longer competent to sign the DNR, your health care proxy or other family member (DNR surrogate) will be able to do so for you.

The DNR form will be given to you at the time of your admission to a hospital or a nursing home in the State of New York. Signing a DNR form does not preclude you from treatment to keep you comfortable and free of pain until the time of natural death. You will continue to receive medications as needed and antibiotics should you develop an infection, unless you refuse them. Copies of existing advance directives—health care proxy, living will, and DNR form—should be given to your family and to your doctor.

---

* The authors thank Judy Ahronheim, M.D. and Felix Silverstone, M.D. for their expert assistance with the key on living wills and DNR (Key 48).

49

DEATH AND AUTOPSY

Why do Alzheimer's victims die? After an average of 10 to 12 years of progressive degeneration, the brain is no longer able to command the body's functions. Sufferers then become unable to walk, to speak, to control bowel and bladder function, or to swallow food. They are at high risk for malnutrition, dehydration, and infection. The most common causes of death are *aspiration pneumonia*, that is, breathing food material and saliva into the lungs rather than swallowing into the stomach, and overwhelming urinary infections. In the end, the individual becomes unresponsive and slips into a peaceful coma.

Discuss with the physician where you prefer to have your loved one die. Many Alzheimer's victims live in and are cared for in the home setting. In small communities, your doctor may come to visit. In larger cities, visiting nurse agencies provide services. If you think that your loved one has expired, the police (911, if available in your area) can be called to your home. The police officer will contact the physician or medical examiner and release the body to the funeral home of your choice. The death certificate is signed later by the physician.

It is a good idea to select the funeral parlor in advance and to have the telephone number available. You should also discuss in advance with your family the kind of religious services that you would like and that you think your loved one would have chosen. Funerals can be very expensive; the time to plan them is not when you are emotionally strained at the time of the death of your loved one. You may not be able to think straight and make wise decisions.

If you would rather have the individual admitted to a health care setting, contact the physician or take the individual to the nearest emergency room. Make sure that the individual's wishes and your own wishes regarding do not resuscitate orders are known to the physician responsible for the admission. In particular, if the individual is already in a nursing home, it is *not* necessary to require transfer to a hospital in the terminal stages. *Acute care settings*—hospitals—should be reserved for those whose outcome can be improved by medical intervention.

As you witness the ultimate deterioration of your loved one, it is wise for you to give strong consideration to an autopsy. Today, the only way to make a definite diagnosis of Alzheimer's disease is by brain biopsy or autopsy. It is very important to you, to your family, and to the scientific world in general to know for sure whether this individual had Alzheimer's disease. It is possible for you to request that only the brain be autopsied. Pathologists are trained to perform skilled organ excision so that no scarring or disfiguration is visible. If you need specific autopsy information, you can call the Alzheimer's Association chapter in your area. They may suggest that you contact a local university center. The advantage of doing this is that these large center programs can often cover the cost of the autopsy without your financial involvement. An autopsy is costly, and insurance does not usually provide reimbursement. Also, university centers are well equipped and well staffed with experienced pathologists who are best able to give you and your physician an accurate diagnosis.

You may want to discuss autopsy with your spiritual advisor. The Judeo-Christian religions permit autopsy if it benefits the surviving relatives. This is also the purpose of Alzheimer's research. By assisting and collaborating with autopsies and research, you may help gather information that leads to the cure for Alzheimer's disease.

50

RESEARCH: THE FUTURE

Although today Alzheimer's disease remains a mystery, the future is promising.

Public attention has been successful in changing health care policy in our nation. The Alzheimer's Association (AA) and the American Association of Retired Persons (AARP) have been instrumental in obtaining federal funds for bio-medical research. In April 1987, the U.S. Congress Office of Technology Assessment issued its report, *Losing a Million Minds: Confronting the Tragedy of Alzheimer's Disease* (Washington, DC). This report also addresses the gaps in Medicare and Medicaid coverage for long-term care. Many elderly people do not realize that Medicare does not cover any of the "custodial" chronic needs of the Alzheimer's victim, such as a home attendant, respite services, or prolonged nursing home costs. The need of the public for a more comprehensive form of health insurance coverage is becoming increasingly obvious. Private sector long-term insurance organizations are involved in developing new appropriate packages that may include tax advantages to defray costs. Thus far, eight states have been successful in developing long-term care insurance for individuals with Alzheimer's disease.

As the country supports Alzheimer's disease research, new advances in scientific areas can be undertaken. In 1991, a record funding of $280 million for Alzheimer's research was voted by the U.S. Congress, with a health spending bill emphasizing the need for better diagnostic technology and drug testing. This amount is twice that allocated for research only two years earlier. Researchers are looking at blood tests for early and more definite identification of Alzheimer's disease and at agents and processes that closely interact with the cause of the degenerative process we call Alzheimer's disease. There are also innovative directions of study and trials for the treatment of Alzheimer's disease. For instance, medications used to improve processes within heart cells may also be useful for brain function. Transplants of healthy young brain cells may be used to replace damaged tissue. Understanding the causes of aging and normal cell death along with the multiple factors leading to cell destruction is essential to unraveling the Alzheimer's mystery.

New procedures for treatment are currently being developed, and researchers are always interested in potential subjects. Contact the university. Find out who is in charge of new treatments for Alzheimer's disease. Discuss the purpose of the study, the criteria for selection, the possible side effects, and the cost, if any, of participation.

It is our fervent hope that the impressive growth in Alzheimer's research nationwide and internationally will lead to a significant breakthrough within the next decade, so our children can live in a world where Alzheimer's disease is a curable or, even better, a preventable illness.

QUESTIONS AND ANSWERS

Q. How do I know if I am getting Alzheimer's disease when I begin to forget people's names?

A. Memory lapses are very common at all ages. Children and young adults forget their homework at school; busy adults forget dental appointments; elderly people forget the names of people they met briefly or have not seen recently. Overwhelmed with a constant flow of information, our minds selectively remember only those details that are essential to our daily activities. These key details vary from one individual to another, depending on our jobs, responsibilities, and families. For instance, a history teacher is bound to remember many more historical dates and events than a computer programmer who has not reviewed social studies in 20 years.

If you keep forgetting things you think you used to remember, ask yourself, first, how important it is for you to remember those specific facts. If it is essential that you remember them, use memory tricks.

Mnemonics is a wonderful tool to assist you to remember people's names. Associate the person's name with a picture or an object. The more unusual or silly the association, the better it strikes you and stays in your mind! For instance, a Ms. Parkinson can be visualized as a lovely "park" with an "inn" and a "son"" ready to bring you a cup of tea.

Other practical tricks to find commonly misplaced objects, such as keys or glasses, can be new keyholders behind your doors or eyeglass chains around your neck. Retrace your own steps if you find yourself entering a room without knowing what you came in for.

If you continue to have trouble with your memory, however, it may be that you are experiencing difficulty in concentrating because you have a lot on your mind or you are depressed. You may want to sit back and think about your personal situation at this point in time. Do you need help? Should you be discussing your concerns with your family or your friends? Should you seek professional advice?

With normal aging, one tends to forget the names of people and lose the ability of abstract reasoning. As a rule, if your judgment is intact and your memory losses intermittent and you feel happy without any tendency to depression, you are probably not developing Alzheimer's disease.

Q. Should I tell my spouse that I have noticed his or her memory loss?
A. Definitely yes. Memory losses can be benign but they can also be the first sign of serious medical problems. Sometimes the problem is treatable and curable. For instance, many depressed individuals manifest memory losses because they have lost interest in life and are no longer concentrating on new information. Therefore, they may repeat a question out of distraction.

Depression is a common illness in later years and responds well to medical treatment. These individuals deserve the benefit of a therapeutic trial of antidepressants.

If the memory loss is in fact due to Alzheimer's disease, it is important that the individual be allowed to plan for his or her own future, the earlier the better. In the early stages, memory is affected but judgment is normal. Your spouse can express his or her wishes and decide now what he or she wants for the future. You can help by arranging a visit to a competent physician as soon as possible.

Q. How does a CAT scan or MRI scan of the brain show Alzheimer's disease?
A. It is a common misunderstanding that CAT or MRI scans "show" Alzheimer's disease. These radiological tests give the physician an image of the brain that is normal in Alzheimer's

disease. The physician wants to make sure that the symptoms are not the result of a brain tumor or a series of strokes or other neurological problems that *would* show up on the scan. New radiological technologies are being developed that show us not only the structure of the brain but also the function. Instead of a photograph, we can now look at a video film! With these technologies, called PET and SPECT scans, the radiologist may be able to see metabolic changes compatible with Alzheimer's disease. However, these tests are not yet widely available.

Q. I have noticed that my mother is having serious memory troubles. She has been living alone in her apartment since my father died 12 years ago. Should I bring her to my home?
A. This is a very delicate situation. You may want to discuss your particular situation with your physician and/or social worker.

As a rule, it is not a good idea to switch environment on a demented elderly person. These individuals may have deeply rooted instincts and environmental clues that allow them to function in their homes despite advanced memory impairment. In a new and different environment, they fall apart. Alzheimer's sufferers may become more confused and more agitated.

In addition, the stress placed on you and your family when you shelter a demented individual in your home is extraordinary. Unless you *and your family* (spouse, children, and other significant relatives) are fully prepared to accept this new responsibility, do not undertake it. It is often impossible to truly anticipate the impact of a new live-in member in the family circle. When that newcomer is demented, the problems may be insurmountable.

Family dynamics are complex at best. What was your relationship with your mother when she was well? What was your husband's relationship with his mother-in-law? How did you take care of his mother or his father when they were ill? How will your children feel about the new situation?

It is better to arrange for support in the individual's home and visit as often as you can possibly manage. Eventually, you may have to consider an institutionalized setting when your mother is no longer aware of her surroundings and has developed physical dysfunctions which make it impossible for you to continue to keep her in the house.

Q. I have kept my father in his home with a good live-in home health attendant. When I visit, he keeps telling me he wants to go home. I don't know what to do.

A. In the advanced stages of the disease, demented persons become disoriented about time, place, and person. They are no longer sure what is "home." Often, they refer to their childhood "home," which no longer exists.

A calm, reassuring approach, pointing to familiar objects and people, is the best approach. If you notice growing anxiety in the repeated need to "go home," it may be time to prescribe anxiety-relieving medications. Discuss this with the treating physician. This need to go home is very disturbing to family members who are working so hard to keep the individual home. Try to understand and accept that no one will be able to re-create the "home" your father is longing for. Don't argue with him. Attempt to distract him by engaging him in another activity, such as a meal or a television show.

Q. My wife has had Alzheimer's disease for eight years, and I have done everything I can to keep her happy. She follows me everywhere, every minute, every day. She even follows me to the bathroom. I am getting older and I am not in good health. What will I do with her if I get sick and need to go to the hospital?

A. You have already taken the first step in the right direction by realizing the precariousness of your situation. It is very important for you to discuss emergency plans for your wife with the physician. Think these plans through now, calmly. Can you count on a child to come and help you? Do you have a supportive neighbor or friend who could move in for a few days? If so, you need to leave an *updated* list of instructions with the name of your physician, medications, when and how to take them, and specific habits (such as milk and cookies at bedtime).

Most cities have crisis centers that provide emergency respite. Get their telephone numbers *now* from the local Alzheimer's Association chapter or the doctor.

If you have absolutely no solution, you can rely on local emergency medical services to bring your spouse to the emergency room of the nearest hospital. Emergency medical services do not take you or your loved one to the hospital of your choice. Keep in mind, however, that most emergency rooms are crowded and busy with true medical crises. This solution should be discouraged and avoided at all costs.

Q. I can handle my spouse's condition the way he is now. Will he get worse, and if so how soon?
A. The individual course of Alzheimer's disease is very unpredictable. In fact, current research indicates that there are probably several types of Alzheimer's disease; in other words, the illness is *heterogeneous*. Some patients get worse very quickly and die within a couple of years. Others progress slowly, and many survive for 10 to 15 years.

We have no scientific data to guide us on how to prolong the life of an Alzheimer's disease sufferer, but a commonsense approach supports good nutrition, plenty of exercise, and intellectual stimulation at an appropriate level.

One thing to keep in mind is to take good care, physically and emotionally, of yourself! You may be in for a long haul. Look for respite care, and treat yourself to enriching hobbies and social activities.

Q. I am so embarrassed when I take my husband to public events. How can I cover up for his memory loss?
A. It is time to reorganize your life for his sake and yours. Public engagements, dinner parties, and business meetings

may be getting to be too much for both of you. A normal conversation requires constant input from memory banks, to identify people's names, roles, family or business relationships, common life events, mutual acquaintances, and so on. Inability to access the memory bank effectively builds frustration and depression. The public function becomes a source of embarrassment for the individual, who eventually gives excuses to avoid them.

The pressure on the spouse is intolerable. There is no way you can manage to control your partner's speech and cover up for his memory losses. Realize that both you and he will feel much more comfortable in a small, friendly group, perhaps limited to close lifelong friends or family members. Explain to these friends that your husband has been diagnosed as having Alzheimer's disease and that they should expect memory lapses in conversation. Reinforce, however, the pleasure that you both have in being able to share their company and enjoy happy moments of togetherness.

Q. My mother gets very angry at times. Could she become dangerous and hurt my children?
A. Because Alzheimer's victims are often depressed and frustrated, they sometimes express anger in the form of spontaneous outbursts of verbal or physical abuse. Not all individuals act out, and many become more docile as time goes on.

However, even when an individual behaves in an aggressive fashion, it is important to remember that their judgment is failing. In other words, an Alzheimer's victim no longer has the ability to develop and execute a plan of action that would include taking a firearm, waiting for the right moment, and shooting a designated victim. In addition, it is extremely unlikely that the individual would injure someone, particularly a child, unless there has been a history of such psychiatric problems. In fact, individuals with Alzheimer's seem to retreat more into themselves as time goes on and become less aware of their surroundings. Learn what triggers the sufferer's agitation. Perhaps it is a loud television show or the music your teenager is blasting throughout the house. Enlist your family's help in suppressing negative stimuli to decrease the likelihood of an outburst. Teach your family to help you in distracting Grandma, and never argue with her.

If you are concerned about a particular behavior, discuss it with your physician. Tranquilizers are available.

Q. I feel so guilty; sometimes I can't handle the stress and I start screaming and yelling at my wife. She has had Alzheimer's disease for five years now. I know she can't help herself. I am afraid I might really hurt her one day.
A. Your situation is very common. It is extraordinarily difficult to cope with an Alzheimer's victim 24 hours a day, 365 days a year. What have you done lately for yourself? What respite have you given yourself? When was your last vacation, away from her? What fun or restful activities have you scheduled for yourself on a weekly basis?

It is essential that you manage to find some time off. No one is expected to work every day without a break. Your work is the most difficult of all.

Ask yourself two questions:
1. Is there any hobby or interest you would like to pursue? Call a nearby recreational center or adult program, and schedule yourself for a class.
2. Would you like to have some time to yourself in your own home, alone? Explore community respite centers, where you can take your wife on a regular basis, or find a neighbor who would watch your wife in her home for a few hours for a prearranged fee. Don't hesitate to spend the money. These are expenses for your own health as well, and you are worth it.

Q. How will I know when it is time for a nursing home?
A. A move to the nursing home is right when either you or the Alzheimer's victim, preferably both of you, are ready for

it. An Alzheimer's victim who no longer recognizes his or her own environment as his or her own home, who no longer recognizes family members and close friends, who requires assistance in the basic activities of daily living, such as bathing, going to the toilet, and eating will probably be just as comfortable in a good nursing facility.

This solution may actually provide you with much needed rest and peace of mind so that you can recharge your batteries. Your visits to the nursing home will become meaningful, peaceful, and useful. You will be able to provide quality time. Try to avoid arriving at the nursing home solution during a crisis. Why not visit a few nursing homes in your area now, so that you become familiar and accustomed to their atmosphere? Be aware that good nursing homes have a waiting list of several months. Even if there is no wait, you will need time to carefully review the financial arrangements and arrange for a down payment.

Q. The doctor told me my father has Alzheimer's disease. How sure can I be that this is the correct diagnosis?
A. The two major causes for progressive, chronic memory loss are Alzheimer's disease and multiple strokes, also called *multiinfarct dementia* (MID). The diagnosis of Alzheimer's disease remains a reasonable opinion based on the best available information. There is no blood test at this point that confirms Alzheimer's disease. The final confirmation is based on an analysis of brain tissue if an autopsy is performed after the patient's death. Very few medical centers consider a brain biopsy on a living patient. Such an invasive procedure is only acceptable if there are reasonable potential benefits.

Studies have been done comparing the accuracy of the physicians' diagnosis based on clinical grounds with the pathologists' confirmation on autopsy. Experienced physicians are correct over 90 percent of the time.

If you are concerned about the accuracy of the diagnosis, discuss with your physician the need for a second opinion in a specialized center, and arrange for an autopsy after your loved one's death. Be sure that you understand how to reach the physician or the pathology department of the hospital on nights and weekends and how to arrange for transportation of the body to the medical center. Also inquire about the costs of a postmortem study. Sometimes, by participating in a research study, you will receive financial support for these expenses.

Q. Is Alzheimer's disease hereditary?
A. Families are generally concerned about the possibility of genetic transmission of Alzheimer's disease. There have been reports of a handful of families in the world in whom the disease is found in each generation and among most siblings, but there is little evidence to support the belief that Alzheimer's disease is hereditary. It can be found in several members of the same family merely because it is a common illness.

Researchers believe that there are probably different types of Alzheimer's disease. The rare familial type of hereditary Alzheimer's disease seems to be transmitted directly from parent to child, affecting both males and females of the same family. It also appears to affect younger individuals, usually in their 40s and 50s.

It is sometimes difficult for family members to know what their aunts, uncles, or grandparents died of, especially if these relatives did not live in the United States. As a rule, if there has been no documented family history of memory problems, your family is unlikely to have a hereditary risk.

Q. Are there medications that work?
A. We need to understand that there are two types of medications: those that work on the illness itself, that is, the memory loss and judgment failure, and those that work on the behavioral symptoms, such as agitation and anxiety.

Q. What types of medication are prescribed for the disease itself?

A. There have been multiple trials of medications based on studies that measured the changes in chemical agents that ease the transmission of information from one nerve cell to another. Because one of these chemical agents, acetylcholine, seems to be reduced in Alzheimer's disease, many researchers have attempted to increase the level of this agent by giving lecithin, the natural substance from which it is formed. Unfortunately, acetylcholine is not utilized effectively by the body when taken by mouth, and circulating blood levels may vary greatly. The results of these trials have not been clearly successful.

Newer drugs, such as Tacrine, which increase the level of acetylcholine indirectly by blocking its decay, have been tested extensively but have still not been approved by the FDA for general use in the community because of reports of liver damage in some patients.

If you are interested in participating in a research study, ask your physician to refer you to an Alzheimer's research center. Remember, however, that most centers do not accept patients in poor physical health or in advanced stages of the disease.

Another long-standing approach has been Hydergine®. Its mechanism of action remains unknown, but many patients and family members believe that it might be of some benefit. Because it has virtually no side effects and is well tolerated, many physicians prescribe it.

Q. What types of medications may be prescribed for the behaviorial symptoms of the disease?

A. There are many good drugs to control agitation, depression, and anxiety. Your physician can help you by prescribing one of these drugs for your loved one. Make sure that you understand the possible side effects of any medication prescribed, particularly the major tranquilizers (Haldol, Mellaril, and Navane) so that you can notify the physician if you observe them. The most troublesome side effect is *tardive dyskinesia*: patients develop involuntary rolling motions of the tongue. This side effect usually reverses if the drug is stopped promptly.

Q. My husband insists on driving the car. At this point, he doesn't even recognize his own children. What do I do?
A. Confronting your spouse who has Alzheimer's disease with the reality that he can no longer drive is a difficult task. To him, driving represents autonomy, freedom, and self-esteem. Giving up driving is giving up control, independence, and usefulness. Often the easiest route for a spouse is to get the family doctor to make the decision and to inform the patient. The patient may forget, however, and go back to his car.

It is your role to remove the car keys from the keyring. Consider selling the car or giving it to one of your children.

Make sure that you request from your physician a sedative or a tranquilizer you can administer if your spouse gets angry.

When your spouse asks you for the car keys or looks for the car, remind him gently that the doctor no longer wants him to drive. You do not need to specify the reason for this decision. Sometimes, it is helpful to have the doctor write "No Driving" on a prescription note, which you can show to your husband.

Explore alternative means of transportation if you do not drive yourself. In many towns, cab companies organize regular pickup services for the supermarket or church. You may also find that a neighbor might be interested in providing some driving in exchange for money or other services.

Q. My husband wakes up in the middle of the night and starts getting dressed to go to work. He has been retired for 18 years. How do I handle this?
A. If your husband has problems sleeping through the night, discuss management of insomnia with your doctor. In general, exercise and activity during the day, coupled with a light

dinner and no caffeine in the evening, should help produce an uninterrupted night. Insist that the individual change into comfortable pajamas that are obviously nightclothes, rather than a T-shirt and underwear.

Sometimes the individual may need a sleeping pill. Tranquilizers at night may be necessary. However, even these medications may not be sufficient.

In the advanced stages of the disease, the Alzheimer's victim may reverse his daily cycle and sleep during the day rather than at night. At this point, you must consider either nursing home placement or a 24-hour home health attendant who can take over for you and give you some respite. Your health and your sleep are very important, not only for you but also for your loved one. If you become sick or burned out, there is no one to assist and care for him.

Do not feel guilty about seeking help at this stage. You are doing the right thing.

If an aide is working at night in your home, allow the aide to stay in your loved one's bedroom while you move to a separate bedroom or a different room. The Alzheimer's sufferer may feel more reassured in his own bed surrounded by familiar furniture.

Q. My mother repeats herself over and over. Do I correct her, or do I go along with it?

A. Repetitions are the hallmark of Alzheimer's disease. Victims repeat themselves often, particularly about items of little perceived importance, such as time of appointments or schedules. Being asked the same question over and over again can drive the caregiver up the proverbial wall. It is natural to attempt to correct someone who is repeating erroneous facts or to stop somebody from restating the same information. The temptation to say, "I told you that already, aren't you listening to me?" is great. Of course, the individual was probably listening but cannot remember what you said.

To prepare yourself for the fact that your mother is about to ask you the same question again, tell yourself that she will do so, so that you begin in some sense to take control of the situation. Also, decide on a standard answer that you can easily repeat while you are carrying on other tasks or other thoughts.

For example, you may have received flowers for your birthday and told your mother with Alzheimer's that your brother sent them to you. Five minutes later, she enters the room and says, "Where did you get these beautiful flowers?" This same question is repeated for the next two hours until you become utterly frustrated. What should you do? Distract her. Change the situation. Either remove the flowers to your bedroom, or remove your mother from the living room by taking her for a walk or for lunch at a fast-food restaurant.

As a general rule, you should never correct or reprimand the Alzheimer's victim. This only causes your mother to feel agitation and anger and guilt on your part. Besides, it is totally useless.

Q. My aunt died yesterday. She and my mother were very close, but my mother has had Alzheimer's disease for the past eight years and I didn't tell her that her sister was ill. Do I tell her that she died?

A. The answer depends on the severity of the disease. If she is in the early stages of the disease, that is, she still recognizes family members and inquires about their health, she should be told that her sister died and be allowed to partake in the grieving process with the family. Contact her physician, and ask if a mild tranquilizer should be prescribed in case of agitation. Also, consider taking along a friendly neighbor or paid companion to the funeral whose role will be to stay at all times by her side.

If your mother is severely demented and has no recollection of family members, there is no need to provoke anxiety, stress, and confusion by reporting the death of a relative.

A difficult exception should be made in the case of the death of a child. In our experience, even very demented individuals may understand when told that a child has died. They should be told the truth with appropriate medical support. However, do not be surprised if the severely demented individual later asks who died or forgets that someone died. This may be a natural and helpful way of denying too painful a reality and finding comfort. In fact, individuals may develop hallucinations and believe that a spouse who died many years ago or a child is with them in the house. Do not attempt to bring them back to reality if they are satisfied with the delusion.

Q. My wife refuses to leave the house. She won't come with me to the movies or to a restaurant. She won't even visit our children. Why? Should I insist that she come?
A. Social withdrawal is part of the dementing process. As a person loses her memory, she develops an awareness and self-consciousness of her inability to remember her friend's names or what happened the week before. Therefore, she attempts to avoid social gatherings in the fear of being confronted with questions she can't answer. At this stage, your wife may make unexpected excuses, such as "I can't go to visit the kids, I have to do my laundry," when you know perfectly well that the laundry can be done tomorrow.

The first step for you is to understand her reaction. It is good for her to remain actively involved in a social group, but you must control and organize the social setting. A highly critical group of bridge players or a sophisticated gathering of business colleagues may no longer be suitable company for your loved one's well-being and self-esteem. Rethink your wife's friends. Who among them are true friends rather than acquaintances? Who can you approach, explain the situation, discuss the medical diagnosis, and ask for understanding support? It may be better for your wife to go out to the movies with only one of her former bridge partners, the one who won't challenge her or criticize her.

Some individuals with Alzheimer's disease have massive denial and do not perceive the extent of the memory impairment. They may insist on continuing their work or their games when their colleagues or friends can no longer tolerate their company. Again, you must take charge and approach the one true friend to escort your wife to more appropriate and less challenging activities.

In the later stages, as the disease progresses, social withdrawal becomes the norm. The brain no longer functions, and the patient cannot respond to the very complex demands of a social gathering. We often hear, "She doesn't want to do anything" or "She just sits there." This is part of the disease and needs to be accepted as such. You need to adjust to this by having your loved one sit quietly in her usual chair while friends and family carry on with the conversation. Do not take the individual to elaborate affairs. Do not expect her to cope with a party atmosphere. Attend small family gatherings where no one will challenge her. Instruct friends and family members, particularly young children, to avoid questions but rather to be friendly and warm and make general statements, such as "I am happy you are here with us," "This is a nice party," or "Here you go, I brought you a sandwich." Prepare your family ahead of time. Tell them to expect repetition and not to react to them.

Q. How far has research progressed? Will there be a cure in the near future?
A. In the last decade, research in Alzheimer's disease has grown more than in the past century. Since 1980, over $1.2 billion has been invested in research for grants in Alzheimer's disease through the U.S. Congress and the National Institutes of Health. Researchers from all over the world are gathering in international conferences to share their findings and explore new avenues.

Research focuses not only on the cause of Alzheimer's disease, that is, possible genetic changes or infections or toxins, but also on the treatment. Medications are available that may be needed in combination to replace those chemicals lost in Alzheimer's disease. It is hoped that these medications may be able to restore function in the brain. Researchers are finding new ways to make sure that the drugs actually reach the brain even though they are given by mouth. This is a very complex field that relies on the input of a wide variety of scientists from molecular biology to psychiatry.

One of the problems holding back progress until recently has been the absence of an animal model. Such a model would be an excellent subject for experimenting and testing medications before trying them on humans. One researcher recently was able to produce a *lesion* (injury) in the brain of a rat. The rat forgets what it was trained to do. This model is now helping us understand the pathology and explore medications that may help.

Unfortunately, the task ahead is arduous and will require years to complete. It is unlikely that we will find a cure within this generation, to treat those individuals who are now victims of the disease. However, the pharmaceutical industry is hopeful that we may soon have drugs to help us in better treating this dreaded illness.

GLOSSARY

Acetylcholine An essential neurotransmitter or chemical substance that allows communication between the brain cells.

Alzheimer, Alois German psychiatrist who first described the disease in 1907 when observing one of his patients, a 51-year-old woman with mental problems.

Amyloid A substance made of protein, which can be found in many organs including the brain and produces a harmful effect on the function of this organ.

Aphasia Inability to speak or to understand speech as a result of brain damage.

Autopsy A detailed examination of a body, involving small samplings of organs for microscopic study, done by a physician after the death of a patient.

CAT scan or CT scan (computerized axial tomography) A series of images obtained by sequential sections of any part of the body performed in a radiologist's office with the use of special x-ray equipment.

Competency A legal term awarded by a judge based on a physician's report of the individual's awareness of his or her situation and the ability to make decisions.

Dementia A global (comprehensive) term to describe a condition in which the mind (*mens*) does not function normally. One of the many possible causes of dementia is Alzheimer's disease.

DNR (do not resuscitate) A document by which you instruct the physician not to perform aggressive measures to attempt to restore a heart beat after your death.

Geriatrics A subspecialty of medicine that specifically studies the medical problems of elderly people.

Gerontology The study of aging in general, not limited to medical knowledge.

Hallucination Perception of a smell, a sound, or an object that is not really present.

Incontinence A physical condition in which the individual can no longer voluntarily control urine (urinary incontinence) or stools (fecal incontinence).

Living will A document that gives your instructions for your medical care in case you become permanently incapacitated.

Mnemonics Techniques used to improve the memory.

MRI (magnetic resonance imaging) A series of images obtained by sequential sections of any part of the body, performed in a radiologist's office using electronic properties in a magnetic field.

Paranoia Unfounded suspicion of people, often expressed as an accusation of stealing money or objects.

Proxy A person designated by you to act on your behalf and make decisions regarding your health care when you are no longer able to do so.

Respite Relief of the burden associated with caring for an Alzheimer's victim. Usually, respite is provided by health care professionals either in the home or in a setting outside the home.

Sedation A relaxed physical and mental state usually produced by taking medications to reduce nervousness and agitation.

Senility The memory loss and general behavioral changes sometimes seen in normal elderly (*senex*) individuals. Originally, senility was used as a synonym for Alzheimer's disease. Physicians now avoid the term because normal aging is not associated with mental illness.

Stroke A medical condition due to a blockage of one or several of the vessels of the brain; often results in paralysis of one side of the body and speech problems.

APPENDIX

ADDITIONAL READING

General

1. Howard Gruetzner. *Alzheimer's: A Caregiver's Guide and Sourcebook.* New York, NY: John Wiley & Sons, 1988.

2. Nancy Mace and Peter Robins, M.D. *The 36-Hour Day.* Baltimore: Johns Hopkins University Press, 1981.

3. Donna Cohen and Carl Eisdorfer. *The Loss of Self: A Family Resource for the Care of Alzheimer's Disease and Related Disorders.* New York, NY: W.W. Norton & Co., 1986.

4. Anne C. Kalick. *Confronting Alzheimer's Disease.* Washington, D.C.: American Association of Homes for the Aging, 1987.

5. Julia Frank. *Alzheimer's Disease: The Silent Epidemic.* Minneapolis: Lerner Publications, 1985.

6. Anthony F. Jorm. *A Guide to the Understanding of Alzheimer's Disease and Related Disorders.* New York: New York University Press, 1987.

7. Lenore Powell and Kate Courtice. *Alzheimer's Disease: A Guide for Families.* Reading, MA: Addison-Wesley, 1983.

8. Miriam K. Aronson. *Understanding Alzheimer's Disease: What It Is, How to Cope with It, Future Directions.* New York, NY: Charles Scribner's Sons, 1988.

9. Steven Zarit, Nancy Orr, and Judy Zarit. *The Hidden Victims of Alzheimer's Disease: Families Under Stress.* New York, NY: New York University Press, 1985.

10. Gail Bernice Holland. *For Sasha, with Love: An Alzheimer's Crusade. The Anne Bashkiroff Story.* New York, NY: Dembner Books, 1985.

11. *Directory of Alzheimer's Disease Treatment Facilities and Home Health Care Programs.* Phoenix, AZ: Orxy Press, 1989.

12. Marion Roach. *Another Name for Madness.* Boston, MA: Houghton Mifflin, 1985.

13. Woodrow Wirsig. *I Love You Too!* New York, NY: M. Evans & Co., 1990.

14. Claire Seymour. *Precipice: Learning to Live with Alzheimer's Disease.* New York, NY: Vantage Press, 1983.

15. William A. Check. *Alzheimer's Disease.* New York, NY: Chelsea House Publishers, 1988.

16. Carmel Sheridan, M.A. *Failure Free Activities for the Alzheimer Patient.* Oakland, CA: Cottage Books, 1988.

17. Joseph L. Matthews. *Eldercare: Choosing and Financing Long-term Care.* Berkeley, CA: Nolo Press, 1990.

18. R. Barker Bausell, M. Rooney, and C. Inlander. *How to Evaluate and Select a Nursing Home.* Redding, MA: A People Medical Society Book, Addison-Wesley Publishing Co., 1988.

19. Jean Crichton. *The Age Care Sourcebook.* A Fireside Book, published by Simon and Schuster, Inc, New York, NY: 1987.

20. Emma Shulman and Gertrude Steinberg. *Caring for an Alzheimer's Disease Patient at Home*. Fidia Parmaceutical Corp, Washington DC, 1988. (Distributed by the New York City Chapter of the Alzheimer's Association, 551 5th Avenue, NY, NY 10176.)

Children's Books

1. Donna Guthrie, in cooperation with the Alzheimer's Disease and Related Disorders Association, Inc. *Grandpa Doesn't Know It's Me*. New York, NY: Human Sciences Press, Inc., 1986.

2. Marsha Kibbey. *My Grammy*. Minneapolis, MN: Carol Rhoda Books, 1988.

3. Judy Delton and Dorothy Tucker. *My Grandma's in a Nursing Home*. Niles, Ill: Tucker, Albert Whitman & Co, 1986.

4. Eric Ruth, *Aunt Dodie has Alzheimer's*. Pentwater, MI; Paraclete, 1988.

5. Doris Sanford. *Maria's Grandma Gets Mixed Up*. In our neighborhood Series. Portland, OR: Multnomah, 1989.

6. Vaunda Micheaux Nelson. *Always Grandma*. New York, NY: G.P. Putnam's Sons, 1988.

7. Mem Fox. *Wilfrid Gordon McDonald Partridge*. A Cranky Nell Book. Brooklyn, NY and La Jolla, CA: Kane/Miller Book Publishers, 1985.

8. Tomie De Paola. *Nana Upstairs and Nana Downstairs*. New York, NY: G.P. Putnam's Sons, 1973.

APPENDIX

COMMUNITY RESOURCES

National Institute on Aging, Information Office Bldg. 31,
Room 5C-36, National Institutes of Health,
Bethesda, MD 20205
Tel 301-496-1752

National Council on the Aging
600 Maryland Avenue, SW Washington, DC 20024
Tel 202-479-1200

Administration on Aging
330 Independence Avenue, S.W.
Washington, DC 20201
Tel 202-619-0724

Alzheimer's Association
70 East Lake Street, Suite 600
Chicago, IL 60601
Tel 1-800-272-3900

Medicare Information
Security Boulevard, Baltimore, MD 21235
Tel 800-772-1213

National Association of Area Agencies on Aging (NAAAA)
1112 16th Street N.W., Suite 100
Washington, DC 20036
Tel 202-296-8130

American Geriatrics Society
770 Lexington Avenue, Suite 300,
New York, NY 10021
Tel 212-308-1414

Asociacion Nacional pro Personas Mayores
(National Association for Hispanic Elderly)
1730 W. Olympic Boulevard
Los Angeles, CA 90015
Tel 213-487-1922

National Indian Council on Aging, Inc.
P.O. Box 2088
Albuquerque, NM 87103
Tel 505-888-3302

American Association of Retired Persons (AARP)
1909 K Street, N.W., Washington, DC 20036
Tel 202-434-2277

National Academy of Elder Law Attorneys, Inc. (NAELA)
655 North Alvernon, Suite 108
Tucson, AZ 85711
Tel 602-881-4005

National Senior Citizens Law Center
1302 18th Street, N.W., Suite 701
Washington, DC 20036
Tel 202-887-5280

Alzheimer's Disease Educational and Referral Center
(ADEAR)
Silver Springs, MD 20907-8250
Tel 301-495-3311

Alzheimer's Family Relief Program
15825 Shady Grove Road, Suite 140
Rockville, MD 20850
Tel 301-948-3244 or 800-437-AHAF
FAX 301-258-9454

Department of Veterans Affairs (VA)
Veterans Health Services and Research Administration
Public Information Office
810 Vermont Avenue, N.W.
Washington, DC 20420
Tel 202-223-2741

ADVANCE DIRECTIVE
Living Will and Health Care Proxy

*D*eath is a part of life. It is a reality like birth, growth and aging. I am using this advance directive to convey my wishes about medical care to my doctors and other people looking after me at the end of my life. It is called an advance directive because it gives instructions in advance about what I want to happen to me in the future. It expresses my wishes about medical treatment that might keep me alive. I want this to be legally binding.

If I cannot make or communicate decisions about my medical care, those around me should rely on this document for instructions about measures that could keep me alive.

I do not want medical treatment (including feeding and water by tube) that will keep me alive if:
- I am unconscious and there is no reasonable prospect that I will ever be conscious again (even if I am not going to die soon in my medical condition), <u>or</u>
- I am near death from an illness or injury with no reasonable prospect of recovery.

I do want medicine and other care to make me more comfortable and to take care of pain and suffering. I want this even if the pain medicine makes me die sooner.

I want to give some extra instructions: [*Here list any special instructions, e.g., some people fear being kept alive after a debilitating stroke. If you have wishes about this, or any other conditions, please write them here.*]

The legal language in the box that follows is a health care proxy. It gives another person the power to make medical decisions for me.

I name _____, who lives at _____

_____, phone number _____,

to make medical decisions for me if I cannot make them myself. This person is called a health care "surrogate," "agent," "proxy," or "attorney in fact." This power of attorney shall become effective when I become incapable of making or communicating decisions about my medical care. This means that this document stays legal when and if I lose the power to speak for myself, for instance, if I am in a coma or have Alzheimer's disease.

My health care proxy has power to tell others what my advance directive means. This person also has power to make decisions for me, based either on what I would have wanted, or, if this is not known, on what he or she thinks is best for me.

If my first choice health care proxy cannot or decides not to act for me, I name _____

_____, address _____,

phone number _____, as my second choice.

(continued on other side)

I have discussed my wishes with my health care proxy, and with my second choice if I have chosen to appoint a second person. My proxy(ies) has(have) agreed to act for me.

I have thought about this advance directive carefully. I know what it means and want to sign it. I have chosen two witnesses, neither of whom is a member of my family, nor will inherit from me when I die. My witnesses are not the same people as those I named as my health care proxies. I understand that this form should be notarized if I use the box to name (a) health care proxy(ies).

Signature _____

Date _____

Address _____

Witness' signature _____

Witness' printed name _____

Address _____

Witness' signature _____

Witness' printed name _____

Address _____

Notary [to be used if proxy is appointed] _____

Drafted and distributed by Choice In Dying, Inc.—the national council for the right to die. Choice In Dying is a national not-for-profit organization which works for the rights of patients at the end of life. In addition to this generic advance directive, Choice In Dying distributes advance directives that conform to each state's specific legal requirements and maintains a national Living Will Registry for completed documents.

CHOICE IN DYING, INC.—
the national council for the right to die
(formerly Concern for Dying/Society for the Right to Die)
200 Varick Street, New York, NY 10014 (212) 366-5540

INDEX

152